NAOMI ALLEN

YOUR GUIDE TO

AGING STRONG

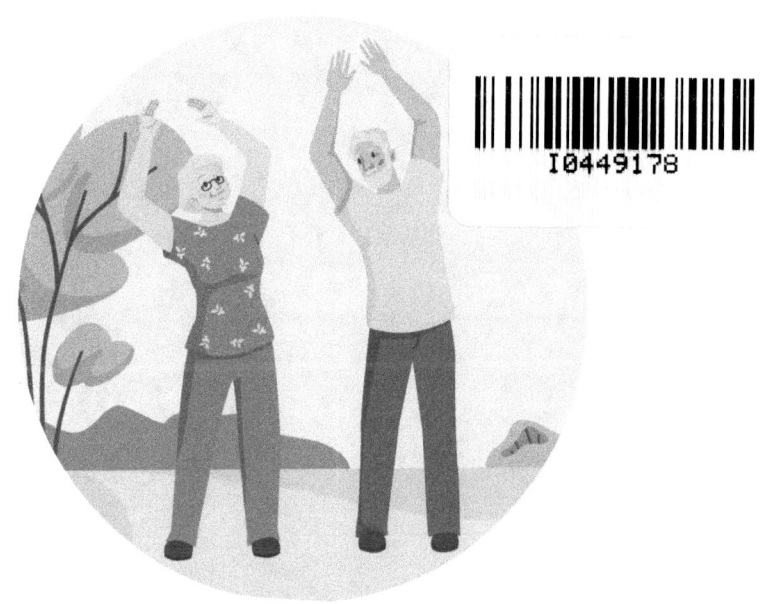

SIMPLE HABITS FOR A
LONGER, HEALTHIER LIFE

Thriving at Every Age

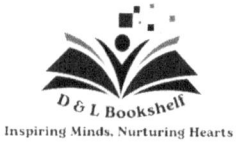

D & L Bookshelf
Inspiring Minds, Nurturing Hearts

Dedication

To those who strive every day to live healthier, happier, and longer lives

This book is dedicated to you. To all the seekers, learners, and doers who understand that every small step toward wellness is a step toward a better future. To all who are embracing the journey of healthy aging with grace, strength, and an open heart—may this book be a source of inspiration, knowledge, and empowerment.

With gratitude,

Naomi Allen

Acknowledgments

A heartfelt thank you to the many researchers, scientists, and health professionals work that has help in the creation of this book, *"Your Guide to Aging Strong: Simple Habits for a Longer, Healthier Life"*. I am deeply indebted. Your commitment to advancing our understanding of health, wellness, and longevity is the foundation upon which this book is built. I hope that my words do justice to your invaluable contributions.

Table of Contents

Bonus Content: (included within chapters)
- 30-Day Movement Challenge:
- 7-Day Longevity Meal Plan
- 10-Day Sleep Improvement Guide
- Gratitude Journal Template
- Long-Term Vision Board Exercise

Introduction

Your Journey to a Longer, Healthier Life

We all share a common desire: to live a long, healthy, and fulfilling life. Yet, many of us are left wondering what exactly we need to do to achieve that goal. We are bombarded with conflicting information from countless sources about what to eat, how to move, and which habits are worth our time and effort. This book is my attempt to cut through the noise and provide you with clear, evidence-based strategies to help you live well and live long.

Why This Book?

In researching the secrets to a longer life, I realized that there isn't a one- size-fits-all solution. Every person's journey is unique, shaped by genetics, lifestyle, and environment. Yet, there are universal principles —grounded in science and proven by the experiences of the world's longest-lived communities—that can guide each of us toward a healthier, more vibrant future. In writing this book, I have drawn from the latest research in aging, nutrition, fitness, sleep, emotional wellness, and stress management. I have distilled this knowledge into practical, actionable steps that you can integrate into your daily routine, regardless of your age or starting point. My goal is to empower you to take control of your health, make informed choices, and cultivate habits that will serve you well for years to come.

What You Will Learn

This book is divided into several chapters, each focusing on a different aspect of healthy aging:

- **Understanding Longevity:** We'll start by exploring the science behind aging and what contributes to a longer life, drawing lessons from those who have lived the longest.
- **Building Daily Habits:** From nutrition and exercise to sleep and emotional wellness, we'll delve into the daily habits that can support your journey to longevity.

- **Personalizing Your Plan:** You'll learn how to create a personalized longevity plan that fits your unique needs and goals, using techniques to stay motivated and overcome obstacles.
- **Leveraging Modern Tools:** We'll discuss how technology and genetic insights can help you tailor your health strategies for optimal results.
- **Managing Stress and Embracing Change:** You'll discover how to manage stress effectively and cultivate resilience, two critical components for a long, healthy life.

A Holistic Approach

This book is not about quick fixes or miracle cures; it's about creating a sustainable lifestyle that promotes health and longevity. By understanding the interplay between different aspects of your well-being—physical, mental, and emotional—you'll be better equipped to make choices that support your goals.

Your Role in This Journey

It's important to remember that longevity isn't just about adding years to your life—it's about adding life to your years. The journey to living well and living long is deeply personal, and the choices you make today will shape your future. Whether you're looking to enhance your energy, prevent disease, or simply feel better day-to-day, the tools and strategies in this book are designed to help you make meaningful progress toward your healthiest, happiest self.

Let's Get Started

I invite you to approach this book with an open mind and a willingness to try new things. Start where you are, take small steps, and celebrate your progress along the way. Remember, the journey to a longer, healthier life is not a sprint—it's a marathon. And with each page you turn, you're taking another step forward. Welcome to your journey to "Your Guide to Aging Strong: Simple Habits for a Longer, Healthier Life".

With warm wishes for your health and happiness,

Naomi Allen

Chapter 1: Longevity Unveiled – Understanding the Science Behind a Long Life

Introduction: A Story of Living Long and Living Well

I remember hearing about Jeanne Calment for the first time—a French woman who lived to be 122 years old, the longest verified human lifespan in history. She wasn't just a remarkable number on a page; she was a living testament to the mysteries of longevity. Jeanne lived independently until the age of 110, still riding her bicycle, eating a diet rich in olive oil, and enjoying her favorite chocolate treats. Her story captivated me, not just because of her age but because of how she lived those years—with vitality, purpose, and joy.

As I delved deeper into her life and the lives of other centenarians, I realized something profound: their stories weren't about secret elixirs or rare genetics. They were about everyday choices—what they ate, how they moved, how they dealt with stress, and how they found meaning in their daily lives. This realization led me on a journey to explore what truly affects how long we live and, more importantly, how well we live those years.

In this chapter, we'll uncover the science behind aging, explore the balance between genetics and lifestyle, and dive into lessons from communities where people regularly live to be 100 or more, the so-called "Blue Zones." My goal is to demystify the path to longevity and show you that a longer, healthier life isn't about radical changes; it's about small, consistent habits that you can start adopting today.

Section 1: The Biology of Aging

To understand how we can live longer, it's essential to start with what's happening inside our bodies as we age. At the cellular level, aging is primarily driven by three key processes: the shortening of telomeres, DNA damage, and oxidative stress. Now, I know these terms might sound a bit like a biology lecture, but bear with me—I'll keep it simple.

Think of your body as a city and your cells as its citizens. Each cell has a nucleus that houses its genetic blueprint, much like a city hall storing essential plans and documents. Telomeres are like the plastic tips on the ends of shoelaces, protecting our chromosomes (the genetic material in our cells) from fraying. Every time a cell divides, these telomeres get a little shorter. Eventually, when they become too short, the cell can no longer divide, leading to aging and, ultimately, cellular death.

Recent studies have shown that telomere length is a reliable indicator of biological age—how old your body feels, regardless of your chronological age. The exciting part? Research suggests that lifestyle choices such as regular exercise, a diet rich in antioxidants, and stress management can help maintain telomere length, effectively slowing down the aging process.

Then there's DNA damage. Imagine if, over time, the blueprints at city hall got smeared with ink or the pages started tearing—this is what happens to our DNA due to factors like UV exposure, pollution, and even normal metabolic processes. Our cells have a robust repair system, but as we age, this system becomes less efficient.

Thankfully, there's good news: studies show that consuming foods high in polyphenols (like berries and dark chocolate) and engaging in activities that boost the body's natural repair processes (like fasting or intermittent fasting) can help reduce DNA damage.

Finally, oxidative stress is another critical player. Picture the city's citizens constantly creating waste that needs to be removed. If the garbage piles up faster than it can be cleared away, the city will start to look and feel rundown. Oxidative stress is the biological equivalent of this garbage buildup—unstable molecules known as free radicals damage cells and tissues, accelerating the aging process. However, incorporating a diet rich in antioxidants, such as leafy greens, nuts, and fruits, and avoiding exposure to pollutants like cigarette smoke, can significantly reduce oxidative stress and protect our cells from damage.

Recent advancements in longevity research, such as the 2023 study published in Nature Medicine, have highlighted the potential for interventions like senolytics, compounds that target and eliminate aging cells, and epigenetic reprogramming, which essentially resets cellular age. While these technologies are promising, the reality is that most of us can significantly impact our aging process by focusing on fundamental lifestyle changes right now.

Section 2: Lifestyle vs. Genetics – The Balancing Act

One of the most common misconceptions about longevity is that it's primarily determined by genetics. "My grandmother lived to be 95, so I'm destined to live long," or "No one in my family makes it past 70, so why should I bother?" These thoughts are understandable but misleading.

Research indicates that genetics account for only about 20-30% of our lifespan. The remaining 70-80% is determined by our lifestyle—our diet, physical activity, sleep, stress management, and social connections. In essence, while our genes provide the framework, our daily habits fill in the details.

Take, for example, the study from Harvard University, which examined identical twins separated at birth. Despite having the same genetic material, their life spans differed significantly based on their lifestyle choices. One twin who ate a balanced diet, exercised regularly, and maintained social connections lived over a decade longer than their sibling who led a more sedentary life with poor dietary habits.

Similarly, a report from the World Health Organization (WHO) suggests that regular physical activity can reduce the risk of chronic diseases like heart disease, stroke, diabetes, and cancer by up to 40%, all of which are significant contributors to premature aging. The WHO also emphasizes that incorporating at least 150 minutes of moderate exercise weekly—like brisk walking or gardening—can add years to one's life.

Lifestyle changes may seem simple, but their impact is profound. It's not about making massive, unsustainable shifts; it's about finding small, manageable changes that fit seamlessly into your daily life. Start by walking an extra 10 minutes each day, swapping out a sugary snack for a handful of nuts, or taking a few minutes to meditate each morning. Over time, these small choices compound, creating a powerful force for longevity.

Section 3: Lessons from the Blue Zones – Habits of the World's Longest-Lived People

When we talk about longevity, we can't ignore the fascinating concept of the "Blue Zones." These are areas where people live significantly longer than the average lifespan, often reaching 100 years or more while maintaining good health and vitality. What's their secret?

The Blue Zones—Okinawa (Japan), Sardinia (Italy), Nicoya (Costa Rica), Icaria (Greece), and Loma Linda (California)—are each unique, but they share common lifestyle traits that we can learn from.

First, consider their diet. People in Blue Zones primarily eat a plant-based diet rich in whole grains, vegetables, fruits, legumes, and nuts. They consume meat sparingly, maybe once or twice a week, and prefer fish. Olive oil is a staple in their kitchens, and they often drink moderate amounts of red wine, which contains heart-healthy resveratrol. These dietary habits align with numerous studies linking plant-based diets to lower risks of heart disease, cancer, and other chronic illnesses.

Movement is another key component. The people in Blue Zones aren't hitting the gym for hours; instead, they incorporate natural movement into their daily routines—walking, gardening, doing household chores, and engaging in community activities. Physical activity is part of their lifestyle, not a scheduled task.

Social connections and purpose play a huge role, too. People in these regions maintain strong social ties with friends, family, and their community. They have a sense of purpose—something to live for, which gives them motivation and meaning every day. Research from the *Journal of Psychosomatic Research* has found that having a purpose in life is associated with a reduced risk of death in older adults.

Lastly, stress management is key. People in Blue Zones practice techniques to reduce and manage stress, such as napping, prayer, meditation, and spending time in nature. Their slower pace of life allows for time to reflect, connect, and rejuvenate, all of which are critical for mental and physical health.

The common thread in these habits? They are all sustainable, simple, and rooted in daily practice. There's no magic bullet or secret formula—just a commitment to living well each day.

Conclusion and Key Takeaways
Longevity isn't about a single secret or a magic pill. It's about a series of small, intentional choices that add up over time. From understanding the biology of aging to recognizing the role of lifestyle over genetics, and learning from the world's longest-lived communities, we see that living longer and healthier is within our control.

Start today by making one small change—take a walk, enjoy a plant-based meal, connect with a loved one, or practice a few minutes of mindfulness. These small steps, repeated daily, will build the foundation for a longer, healthier life.

Remember, the journey to living well and living long begins with a single step. Let's take it together.

Bonus Content: Quick Longevity Self-Assessment

To kickstart your journey toward longevity, take a moment to assess your current habits:

- **Physical Activity**: Do you engage in at least 150 minutes of moderate exercise each week?

- **Diet:** Is your diet primarily plant-based, with minimal processed foods and sugars?

- **Sleep:** Are you getting 7-9 hours of quality sleep each night?

- **Stress Management:** Do you have regular practices to reduce stress, such as meditation or time in nature?

- **Social Connections:** Are you maintaining strong relationships with family and friends?

- **Purpose:** Do you have a clear sense of purpose or goals that motivate you daily?

Scoring:

- Give yourself 1 point for each "Yes" answer.

Results:

- **5-6 Points:** You're on a great path to longevity! Keep up these healthy habits and continue making small improvements.

- **3-4 Points:** You're doing well, but there are some areas for growth. Identify one habit you can focus on improving this week.

- **0-2 Points:** It's never too late to start! Pick one area to focus on first, and remember that even small changes can lead to big results over time.

Use this self-assessment as a starting point to reflect on your current lifestyle and pinpoint areas for improvement. Remember, the goal isn't perfection but progress—one small step at a time toward a longer, healthier life

Chapter 2: The Power of Movement – How Moving Your Body Fuels Longevity

Introduction: The Life-Changing Impact of Movement

I'll never forget meeting Marjorie, a sprightly 96-year-old who had more energy than some people half her age. When I asked her secret, she simply smiled and said, "Keep moving." Every morning, Marjorie walks around her neighborhood, rain or shine, for at least 30 minutes. She gardens, does yoga, and even participates in a local dance class. For Marjorie, movement isn't a chore; it's a way of life. Her routine keeps her mentally sharp, physically strong, and emotionally vibrant.

Science backs up what Marjorie intuitively knows. A recent study published in the *British Journal of Sports Medicine* found that just 11 minutes of moderate exercise a day can significantly lower the risk of early death. Another landmark study from the *Harvard Alumni Health Study* revealed that people who engage in regular physical activity have a 25-35% lower risk of death than sedentary individuals. Movement is one of the most potent tools we have to extend our lifespan and improve the quality of those extra years.

In this chapter, we'll explore why regular movement is so vital for longevity. We'll dive into the benefits of different types of exercise, and how even small changes in your daily routine can add years to your life. Remember, the goal isn't perfection; it's progress. And every step, stretch, and squat counts.

Section 1: The Benefits of Regular Movement

Movement is more than just burning calories or building muscles; it's the foundation for a long, healthy life. Here's why:

Physical Benefits: Regular movement significantly reduces the risk of developing chronic diseases. For instance, research from the American Heart Association shows that physical activity can lower the risk of heart disease—the leading cause of death globally—by up to 30%. Exercise also helps manage weight, reduces blood pressure, and improves cholesterol levels, all of which are critical factors in preventing cardiovascular diseases.

Beyond the heart, exercise strengthens bones, improves joint flexibility, and enhances overall muscle function. Weight-bearing activities like walking, jogging, and resistance training have been shown to increase bone density, reducing the risk of osteoporosis and fractures as we age. A study from the Journal of Bone and Mineral Research found that postmenopausal women who engaged in regular weight-bearing exercises had significantly higher bone density than their sedentary peers.

Cognitive Benefits: Physical activity is also a brain booster. Exercise increases blood flow to the brain, promotes the growth of new neurons, and enhances the release of chemicals that protect the brain from age-related decline.

According to a study from the University of British Columbia, regular aerobic exercise appears to increase the size of the hippocampus, the part of the brain involved in memory and learning.

Additionally, a 2023 report published in *The Lancet* highlighted that exercise reduces the risk of developing dementia by up to 30%. Physical activity has been linked to slower rates of cognitive decline and lower incidences of Alzheimer's disease. The message is clear: if you want to keep your brain sharp and your memory intact as you age, make movement a non-negotiable part of your daily routine.

Emotional Benefits: The benefits of regular movement extend beyond the physical and cognitive—they also profoundly impact emotional well-being. Exercise has been shown to release endorphins, the body's natural "feel-good" chemicals, which reduce stress, anxiety, and depression. A large-scale study in *JAMA Psychiatry* found that even small doses of physical activity can lower the risk of depression, highlighting the mental health benefits of regular movement.

Movement also improves sleep quality, which is closely linked to emotional health. A study in the *Sleep Medicine Reviews* journal demonstrated that moderate exercise, such as brisk walking, can help people fall asleep faster, stay asleep longer, and experience deeper, more restorative sleep.

Regular movement truly is a holistic medicine that benefits the body, mind, and soul. It's about more than just extending life; it's about enhancing the quality of those extra years.

Section 2: Types of Movement for Longevity

Now that we've explored the benefits of movement, let's delve into the different types of exercises that can help you live a longer, healthier life. The good news? You don't have to run marathons or lift heavy weights to reap the benefits. A variety of movement types can support longevity, each offering unique benefits:

Aerobic Exercise: Also known as cardio, aerobic exercise includes activities like walking, jogging, cycling, swimming, and dancing. These exercises elevate your heart rate and increase oxygen flow throughout your body, improving cardiovascular health. A study from the *European Heart Journal* showed that engaging in at least 150 minutes of moderate aerobic activity per week reduces the risk of cardiovascular diseases by up to 35%.

But aerobic exercise doesn't just benefit the heart. It also boosts lung capacity, improves circulation, and enhances metabolic function, helping to maintain a healthy weight and prevent conditions like type 2 diabetes. Importantly, research suggests that aerobic exercise can even slow the biological aging process by preserving telomere length, a key indicator of cellular aging.

Strength Training: As we age, we naturally lose muscle mass —a process known as sarcopenia—which can lead to frailty, reduced mobility, and a higher risk of falls. Strength training, which includes activities like weightlifting, resistance band exercises, and bodyweight exercises (like squats and push-ups), is crucial for combating muscle loss and maintaining functional independence.

A study published in the **Journal of Aging and Physical Activity** found that individuals who engaged in regular strength training had better mobility, balance, and overall physical function compared to those who did not. Moreover, strength training has been shown to improve bone density, support healthy metabolic function, and reduce the risk of chronic conditions such as osteoporosis and arthritis.

Flexibility and Balance Training: Often overlooked, flexibility and balance exercises are essential for maintaining mobility and preventing falls—one of the leading causes of injury among older adults. Practices like yoga, tai chi, and Pilates enhance flexibility, improve joint health, and strengthen stabilizing muscles, all of which contribute to better balance and coordination.

A 2022 study in the *Journal of Gerontology* highlighted that older adults who practiced yoga or tai chi regularly experienced fewer falls and improved overall stability compared to those who did not. Furthermore, these practices offer additional benefits for mental health, including reduced stress and anxiety levels, contributing to overall well-being.

By incorporating a mix of aerobic, strength, and flexibility exercises, you can create a balanced movement routine that supports every aspect of your health and longevity.

Section 3: Integrating Movement into Daily Life

It's easy to think that movement means spending hours in the gym, but that's not the case. The key is consistency, not perfection, and integrating movement into your daily routine can be simpler than you think.

Start Small, Build Gradually: Begin with small changes that fit seamlessly into your lifestyle. Take the stairs instead of the elevator, walk or bike to nearby places instead of driving, or do a quick 5-minute stretch routine every morning. These little bursts of activity can add up throughout the day.

Make Movement Enjoyable: Find activities you love, whether it's dancing, hiking, playing tennis, or gardening. The more you enjoy the activity, the more likely you are to stick with it. Research shows that finding joy in movement leads to more consistent exercise habits, which are crucial for long-term health.

Incorporate Movement into Work: If you have a sedentary job, consider strategies like standing desks, walking meetings, or short, regular breaks to stretch and move. Even 5-10 minutes of movement every hour can offset the risks of prolonged sitting.

A study published in the *American Journal of Epidemiology* found that breaking up sitting time with short bouts of movement can lower the risk of premature death by up to 30%.

Create a Routine: Set specific times in your day for movement. Maybe it's a morning walk, a lunchtime yoga session, or an evening strength workout. Consistency is key, so find a routine that works for you and stick to it as much as possible.

Use Technology: Fitness trackers, apps, and online classes can provide motivation, accountability, and structure. Many people find that tracking their steps or setting daily movement goals helps them stay on course.

Involve Others: Movement can be more enjoyable with company. Invite friends or family members to join you in your exercise routine. Join a local fitness class, walking group, or sports team to make new connections and stay motivated.

Conclusion and Key Takeaways

The power of movement in enhancing longevity is undeniable. It benefits every part of our being—our bodies, brains, and emotions. But remember, it's not about intense workouts or grueling schedules; it's about making small, sustainable changes that become a regular part of your life.

Start where you are. If you're new to exercise, begin with a few minutes of walking each day. If you're already active, try incorporating different types of movement for a more balanced routine. The key is consistency and enjoyment.

Moving your body is one of the most powerful tools you have to increase your lifespan and the quality of those years. As you begin to integrate more movement into your daily life, you'll likely find that not only do you feel better physically, but you also feel more energized, focused, and emotionally balanced.

Bonus Content: 30-Day Movement Challenge

To help you get started, here's a 30-day movement challenge designed to gradually build your fitness and seamlessly integrate movement into your daily routine. This challenge focuses on small, consistent steps to create lasting habits.

Week 1: Start Small, Build Consistency
1. **Day 1:** Walk for 10 minutes at a comfortable pace.
2. **Day 2**: Stretch for 5 minutes in the morning and before bed.
3. **Day 3:** Walk for 15 minutes and add 5 squats.
4. **Day 4:** Try a 5-minute dance or aerobic routine of your choice.
5. **Day 5:** Walk for 20 minutes, focusing on your posture.
6. **Day 6:** Do a gentle yoga or stretching session for 10 minutes.
7. **Day 7:** Rest day. Reflect on how these small movements felt.

Week 2: Add Variety and Build Strength

1. **Day 8:** Walk for 20 minutes, incorporating 3 intervals of brisk walking.
2. **Day 9:** Perform 10 squats, 5 lunges per leg, and 10 push-ups.
3. **Day 10**: Try a new activity like cycling or swimming for 15 minutes.
4. **Day 11:** Walk for 25 minutes, adding 5 minutes of brisk walking.
5. **Day 12:** Focus on flexibility: stretch major muscle groups for 15 minutes.
6. **Day 13:** Strength day: 3 sets of 10 squats, lunges, and push-ups.
7. **Day 14:** Rest or active recovery with gentle stretching or a slow walk.

Week 3: Increase Intensity and Enjoyment

1. **Day 15:** Walk for 30 minutes with 5 intervals of brisk walking.
2. **Day 16:** Attend a fitness class or try an online workout.
3. **Day 17:** Strength day: Add resistance with light weights or resistance bands.
4. **Day 18**: Balance and flexibility: Practice yoga or tai chi for 20 minutes.
5. **Day 19:** Walk or hike in a different location for 30 minutes.
6. **Day 20:** Strength day: Focus on core exercises (planks, sit-ups) for 10 minutes.
7. **Day 21:** Rest day or enjoy a leisurely activity like gardening or playing with pets.

Week 4: Challenge Yourself and Reflect

1. **Day 22:** Walk for 35 minutes, incorporating stairs or hills.
2. **Day 23:** High-intensity interval training (HIIT) for 10-15 minutes.
3. **Day 24**: Strength day: Full-body workout with weights or resistance bands.
4. **Day 25:** Flexibility and mindfulness: Longer yoga session (30 minutes).
5. **Day 26:** Try a new sport or physical activity (tennis, martial arts, etc.).
6. **Day 27:** Active play or outdoor adventure (biking, kayaking, etc.).
7. **Day 28:** Rest day or active recovery with light stretching or meditation.

Final Days: Consolidate Your Routine

1. **Day 29**: Walk or jog for 40 minutes at your own pace.
2. **Day 30**: Reflect on the month: Write down how you feel, what changes you've noticed, and set goals for continuing your movement journey.

Reflection and Goal Setting

Ask Yourself:

- How did your body feel after each activity?
- Which types of movement did you enjoy the most?
- What challenges did you face, and how did you overcome them?

Set Future Goals:

- Choose at least three activities from this challenge that you want to continue regularly.
- Set a weekly schedule to maintain consistency.
- Find a movement buddy or group for support and motivation.

By incorporating a variety of movements—cardio, strength training, flexibility, and balance—into your daily routine, you'll not only build a habit of regular exercise but also lay the foundation for a healthier, longer life. Remember, the key to longevity isn't about perfection; it's about persistence and enjoying the journey.

Chapter 3: Nutrition for Longevity – Eating for a Longer Life

Introduction: The Role of Nutrition in Longevity

Imagine a bustling village in Okinawa, Japan, where centenarians are not rare but common. Here, people live well into their 90s and beyond, maintaining health and vitality with ease. Their secret? Nutrition plays a central role. In fact, researchers have found that their plant-based diet, rich in vegetables, legumes, and seafood, contributes significantly to their remarkable longevity. It's not just in Okinawa; across other Blue Zones—regions with the highest number of centenarians—the same patterns emerge.

Recent studies, like the one published in *The Lancet* in 2023, highlight that diet is a leading factor in determining how long and how well we live. The foods we eat influence every aspect of our health: they regulate our metabolism, maintain our immune system, protect against chronic diseases, and even affect our cognitive function. As you will discover in this chapter, nutrition is much more than fuel; it is the foundation upon which a long, healthy life is built.

Let's delve deeper into what a longevity-focused diet looks like, clear up some common misconceptions about so-called "miracle" diets, and explore practical habits you can adopt without turning your life upside down.

Section 1: The Longevity Diet

When we think of a diet that promotes longevity, it's not about deprivation or strict rules. Instead, it's about choosing nutrient-dense, whole foods that nourish the body and mind. Let's break down the components of a diet that can help you live longer and better:

Plant-Based Foods: One of the common denominators in the diets of those living in Blue Zones is a heavy emphasis on plant-based foods. This includes vegetables, fruits, legumes, whole grains, nuts, and seeds. A study published in *The American Journal of Clinical Nutrition* showed that individuals who ate at least five servings of fruits and vegetables per day had a 31% lower risk of mortality compared to those who consumed fewer servings.

Plant-based foods are rich in fiber, vitamins, minerals, and antioxidants—all crucial for combating inflammation and oxidative stress, two key contributors to aging. For example, leafy greens like spinach and kale are packed with vitamins A, C, and K, which support cellular health and boost immune function. Berries, rich in antioxidants, protect cells from damage caused by free radicals. Legumes like beans, lentils, and chickpeas provide protein, fiber, and important micronutrients that support heart health and longevity.

Healthy Fats: Not all fats are created equal. Diets that promote longevity are rich in healthy fats, particularly those found in olive oil, avocados, nuts, and fatty fish like salmon. These fats contain omega-3 fatty acids, which are known for their anti-inflammatory properties and heart health benefits. A study from the Journal of the American Heart Association found that individuals who consumed high levels of omega-3 fatty acids had a 20% lower risk of dying from any cause.

Olive oil, a staple in the Mediterranean diet, is especially noteworthy. It's packed with monounsaturated fats, which help reduce bad cholesterol levels and improve heart health. The *PREDIMED* study, a large-scale research project on the Mediterranean diet, showed that participants who consumed extra-virgin olive oil regularly had a 30% lower risk of heart disease.

Lean Proteins: While plant-based proteins should make up the majority of your diet, lean animal proteins like fish, poultry, and eggs can also play a role. Fish, in particular, is a cornerstone of many longevity diets. Rich in omega-3 fatty acids, fish like salmon, sardines, and mackerel help reduce inflammation and lower the risk of heart disease and cognitive decline. The *Nurses' Health Study* and the Health Professionals Follow-Up Study found that replacing red meat with fish or poultry reduced mortality rates by up to 20%.

Whole Grains and Legumes: Whole grains like quinoa, brown rice, and oats are high in fiber, vitamins, and minerals. They help maintain stable blood sugar levels, support digestive health, and reduce the risk of cardiovascular diseases. A meta-analysis published in the **British Medical Journal** in 2022 revealed that individuals who consume three servings of whole grains daily have a 20% lower risk of developing heart disease, stroke, and type 2 diabetes.

Actionable Tips to Transition to a Longevity Diet:

- **Start small:** Begin by adding one or two servings of vegetables to your meals each day.
- **Swap out**: Replace refined grains with whole grains—try brown rice instead of white, or whole-grain bread instead of white bread.
- **Embrace healthy fats:** Use olive oil for cooking, add avocado to your salads, or snack on a handful of nuts.
- **Prioritize lean proteins:** Replace some of your red meat intake with fish or legumes.
- **Experiment with plant-based meals:** Try going plant-based one day a week with dishes like lentil soup, vegetable stir-fry, or a chickpea salad.

By gradually incorporating these elements, you'll be setting a solid foundation for longevity without overwhelming yourself with drastic changes.

Section 2: Myths and Misconceptions

In the world of nutrition, myths and misconceptions are rampant. Let's debunk some of the most common ones:

Myth: You need a restrictive diet to live longer.
Many people believe that strict diets—like eliminating entire food groups or fasting for long periods—are the keys to longevity. However, studies show that overly restrictive diets can be unsustainable and may lead to nutritional deficiencies. The real secret is moderation. In the Blue Zones, people enjoy a varied diet that includes small amounts of meat, dairy, and even wine. The key is balance and portion control, not restriction.

Myth: You must eat "superfoods" to achieve longevity.
The term "superfood" is often used to market certain foods as miracle cures, but the truth is that there's no single food that will make you live longer. While foods like kale, quinoa, and blueberries are undoubtedly healthy, a diet based on a variety of whole, minimally processed foods is more beneficial. As research suggests, it's the overall pattern of eating that matters most, not specific foods.

Myth: High-protein diets are best for aging.
 High-protein diets, particularly those that rely heavily on animal proteins, have been touted as the best for maintaining muscle mass and overall health as we age.

However, studies, such as one from the Cell Metabolism journal, suggest that while protein is important, excessive animal protein intake may increase the risk of certain diseases, including cancer and heart disease. A balanced approach, emphasizing plant-based proteins like beans, lentils, and nuts, provides the necessary nutrients without the potential risks associated with high meat consumption.

Myth: Carbs are the enemy.
Carbohydrates have been demonized in recent years, but not all carbs are created equal. Refined carbs (like white bread, pastries, and sugary cereals) can indeed spike blood sugar and contribute to health problems. However, complex carbs found in whole grains, fruits, and vegetables are vital sources of energy, fiber, and essential nutrients. These are the types of carbs found in the diets of the longest-lived populations.

By understanding these myths, you can make more informed choices about your diet and focus on what truly matters for longevity—balance, variety, and moderation.

Section 3: Easy-to-Adopt Eating Habits

Making dietary changes doesn't have to be overwhelming or drastic. Here are some practical habits to help you eat for longevity without upending your entire lifestyle:

Mindful Eating: Slow down and savor each bite. Mindful eating has been shown to improve digestion, reduce overeating, and enhance the enjoyment of food.

Take time to chew thoroughly, notice the flavors and textures, and be present during your meals.

Research from Harvard Health suggests that mindful eating can help reduce calorie intake and support weight management.

Meal Prepping: Set aside a day each week to prepare and portion out meals. This not only saves time but also ensures you have healthy, home-cooked meals ready to go, reducing the temptation to opt for processed or fast food. You could start with something simple, like preparing a big batch of vegetable soup or roasting a variety of veggies and proteins.

Portion Control: Instead of eliminating foods, focus on controlling portion sizes. Use smaller plates, serve yourself smaller portions, and listen to your hunger cues. Studies show that people who are mindful of portion sizes tend to consume fewer calories overall, without feeling deprived.

Incorporate More Whole Foods: Gradually replace processed snacks with healthier options. Swap chips and cookies for nuts, fruits, or yogurt. Keep fresh fruit and vegetables within easy reach and try to include at least one serving of fruits or vegetables in every meal.

Stay Hydrated: Drinking enough water is essential for overall health. Sometimes, thirst can be mistaken for hunger, leading to unnecessary snacking. Aim for at least 8 glasses of water a day and consider drinking a glass before each meal to help control appetite.

By integrating these simple habits into your routine, you can improve your diet without feeling overwhelmed or deprived.

Conclusion and Key Takeaways

The role of nutrition in longevity is undeniable. What we eat not only affects how long we live but also how well we live those years. Adopting a longevity diet—rich in plant-based foods, healthy fats, lean proteins, and whole grains—while avoiding common dietary pitfalls can have a profound impact on our health and lifespan. Remember, it's not about drastic changes or following restrictive diets; it's about making small, sustainable adjustments that you can maintain over the long term.

As you start your journey toward a healthier, longer life, focus on incorporating more plant-based meals, being mindful of portion sizes, and finding joy in the foods that nourish you. Celebrate progress over perfection and know that every healthy choice you make today is an investment in your future self.

Bonus Content: 7-Day Longevity Meal Plan

To help you get started on your journey toward better nutrition, here's a simple 7-day meal plan designed with longevity in mind. These recipes are easy to prepare, nutritious, and delicious:

Day 1:
- **Breakfast**: Overnight oats with chia seeds, almond milk, berries, and a drizzle of honey.
- **Lunch:** Mixed greens salad with quinoa, chickpeas, cucumber, tomato, olive oil, and lemon dressing.
- **Dinner:** Baked salmon with roasted asparagus and sweet potato wedges.

Day 2:
- **Breakfast:** Green smoothie with spinach, banana, Greek yogurt, flaxseed, and a splash of orange juice.
- **Lunch:** Lentil soup with carrots, celery, and tomatoes, served with a side of whole grain bread.
- **Dinner:** Stir-fried tofu with broccoli, bell peppers, snap peas, and brown rice.

Day 3:
- **Breakfast:** Avocado toast on whole grain bread with cherry tomatoes and a poached egg.
- **Lunch:** Chickpea and vegetable wrap with hummus, spinach, bell peppers, and a whole grain tortilla.
- **Dinner:** Grilled chicken breast with quinoa, sautéed spinach, and mushrooms.

Day 4:
- **Breakfast:** Greek yogurt topped with walnuts, blueberries, and a drizzle of maple syrup.
- **Lunch:** Mediterranean bowl with brown rice, roasted vegetables, feta cheese, and tahini dressing.
- **Dinner:** Vegetable curry with cauliflower, chickpeas, tomatoes, and coconut milk, served over jasmine rice.

Day 5:
- **Breakfast:** Scrambled eggs with spinach, tomatoes, and a slice of whole grain toast.
- **Lunch:** Salad with mixed greens, avocado, black beans, corn, cherry tomatoes, and cilantro-lime dressing.
- **Dinner:** Spaghetti with whole grain pasta, marinara sauce, and a side of steamed broccoli.

Day 6:
- **Breakfast:** Smoothie bowl with blended banana, strawberries, almond milk, topped with granola and fresh fruits.
- **Lunch:** Sweet potato and black bean chili served with a side of whole-grain tortilla chips.
- **Dinner:** Shrimp stir-fry with snap peas, bell peppers, garlic, and brown rice.

Day 7:
- **Breakfast:** Whole grain pancakes with fresh berries and a dollop of Greek yogurt.
- **Lunch:** Buddha bowl with brown rice, roasted chickpeas, avocado, cucumber, and tahini sauce.
- **Dinner:** Grilled fish tacos with cabbage slaw, avocado, and a side of mango salsa.

These meals are designed to be both satisfying and nutrient-dense, providing your body with the vitamins, minerals, and antioxidants it needs to thrive. Feel free to mix and match recipes based on your preferences and availability of ingredients. Remember, the goal is to enjoy what you eat while fueling your body for a longer, healthier life.

By making these small, consistent changes to your diet, you'll be on your way to enjoying the benefits of a longevity-focused lifestyle.

Chapter 4: Sleep and Longevity – How Rest Recharges Your Life Span

Introduction: The Crucial Role of Sleep

A few years ago, I met a man named James, a hard-charging executive who prided himself on getting by with only four hours of sleep a night. "I'll sleep when I'm dead," he would joke, often boasting about how his busy schedule left little time for rest. But it wasn't long before James's lack of sleep started catching up with him. He began to notice that his memory was slipping, his energy was dwindling, and he was increasingly irritable. Eventually, he faced a series of health scares that forced him to rethink his relationship with sleep.

James's story isn't unique. A groundbreaking study from the *Centers for Disease Control and Prevention* found that one in three adults in the United States does not get enough sleep, defined as less than seven hours per night. The consequences of poor sleep are well-documented: increased risk of chronic conditions such as heart disease, diabetes, depression, and even early mortality.

But the opposite is also true. Just as inadequate sleep can shorten your life, getting enough high-quality rest can help you live longer and healthier. Sleep is more than just downtime; it's a critical period for the body to repair, restore, and rejuvenate. In this chapter, we'll explore the science behind sleep, discuss practical ways to improve sleep quality, and examine how good sleep habits are essential for longevity.

Section 1: The Science of Sleep

Sleep is a complex and dynamic process that profoundly impacts our brain, body, and overall wellness. To understand its importance, think of sleep as the "night shift" for your body—a dedicated time when essential maintenance, repairs, and clean-up occur.

Sleep and Brain Health: Imagine your brain as a busy city. During the day, it processes an enormous amount of information, akin to city traffic. Sleep is the city's night crew, clearing away debris and fixing damage. The brain uses sleep to consolidate memories, remove toxins, and prepare for the next day's cognitive demands. A study from the *National Institute of Neurological Disorders and Stroke* found that during sleep, the brain's glymphatic system—its waste clearance pathway—works 60% more efficiently, flushing out neurotoxins that build up during waking hours. This process is critical for preventing neurodegenerative diseases such as Alzheimer's.

Cellular Repair and Immune Function: Sleep is also crucial for cellular repair and immune function. Think of your cells as tiny factories constantly working to keep you alive. When you sleep, these factories switch into repair mode, fixing damaged DNA and rebuilding tissues. The body produces most of its growth hormone during deep sleep, which is vital for repairing muscles, tissues, and bones. Moreover, sleep helps regulate the immune system by promoting the production of cytokines, proteins that help fight infections and inflammation. A lack of sleep, therefore, weakens your body's defenses and can make you more susceptible to illness.

Overall Wellness: Sleep impacts nearly every aspect of health and wellness. It regulates hormones, particularly those that control hunger and stress, such as ghrelin, leptin, and cortisol. Poor sleep disrupts these hormones, leading to increased appetite, cravings for high-calorie foods, and weight gain, which can contribute to a range of chronic conditions like obesity, diabetes, and heart disease. Sleep is also essential for emotional health, as it plays a key role in regulating mood and stress responses. Research from the American Psychological Association has shown that inadequate sleep can significantly increase the risk of anxiety, depression, and other mental health disorders.

Understanding the science of sleep reveals just how vital it is to overall health and longevity. It is not a luxury but a necessity that keeps our bodies and minds functioning optimally.

Section 2: Improving Sleep Quality

Now that we understand the critical role of sleep, the question is: how do we improve it? Here are some practical, science-backed strategies to enhance your sleep hygiene:

Establish a Bedtime Routine: A consistent bedtime routine helps signal to your body that it's time to wind down. Try to go to bed and wake up at the same time every day, even on weekends. This routine helps regulate your body's internal clock, or circadian rhythm, which controls sleep-wake cycles. Activities such as reading a book, taking a warm bath, or practicing gentle yoga can help relax your body and prepare your mind for sleep.

Create a Sleep-Friendly Environment: Your bedroom should be a sanctuary for sleep. Make it cool, dark, and quiet. According to the *National Sleep Foundation*, the optimal sleep environment is around 65°F (18°C). Consider using blackout curtains to block out light, earplugs or a white noise machine to drown out noise, and a comfortable mattress and pillows that support restful sleep.

Limit Exposure to Light: Light exposure, especially blue light from screens, can interfere with melatonin production, the hormone that helps regulate sleep. Avoid screens—like phones, computers, and televisions—for at least an hour before bed. Instead, consider reading a physical book, listening to calming music, or practicing relaxation techniques.

Mind Your Diet and Hydration: Avoid heavy meals, caffeine, and alcohol close to bedtime. Caffeine is a stimulant that can disrupt sleep even hours after consumption, while alcohol might make you sleepy initially but can lead to fragmented sleep. Drinking a calming herbal tea, like chamomile or valerian root, may help relax the body and prepare for rest.

Incorporate Relaxation Techniques: Techniques like mindfulness meditation, deep breathing exercises, or progressive muscle relaxation can help calm the mind and prepare the body for sleep. Research from the *Journal of Sleep Research* indicates that mindfulness practices can significantly improve sleep quality and duration by reducing stress and anxiety.

Exercise Regularly: Regular physical activity can promote better sleep, particularly if done earlier in the day. A study from the *Sleep Medicine Reviews* found that people who exercise regularly fall asleep faster, sleep more deeply, and wake up less frequently during the night. Aim for at least 30 minutes of moderate exercise, such as walking or cycling, but try to avoid vigorous exercise close to bedtime as it can have a stimulating effect.

Limit Naps: While short naps can be refreshing, long or irregular napping during the day can negatively affect your nighttime sleep. If you need to nap, try to keep it under 30 minutes and avoid napping late in the afternoon.

Use Sleep Aids Sparingly: While some may find occasional use of sleep aids helpful, it's crucial to use them sparingly and under a doctor's supervision. Over-reliance on sleep medications can lead to dependence and may not address the underlying causes of sleep issues.

By incorporating these habits into your daily routine, you can improve your sleep quality and support your body's natural processes for healing, restoration, and rejuvenation.

Section 3: The Connection Between Sleep and Longevity

The connection between good sleep and longevity is well-established in scientific literature. Research shows that quality sleep contributes to a longer, healthier life in several ways:

Reduced Risk of Chronic Diseases: Studies have consistently shown that poor sleep is associated with an increased risk of chronic diseases. For example, a study published in the *Journal of the American Heart Association* found that people who slept less than six hours per night had a 48% increased risk of developing or dying from heart disease. Similarly, research from the *Harvard T.H. Chan School of Public Health* indicates that inadequate sleep is a significant risk factor for type 2 diabetes, obesity, and certain cancers.

Enhanced Cognitive Function and Brain Health: Good sleep is essential for maintaining cognitive function as we age. Research from the *University of California, Berkeley* found that sleep deprivation contributes to the buildup of beta-amyloid, a protein associated with Alzheimer's disease. Conversely, adequate sleep supports the brain's ability to consolidate memories, process information, and maintain mental acuity. Older adults who maintain good sleep habits are less likely to experience cognitive decline and dementia.

Improved Immune Function: Sleep plays a critical role in supporting the immune system. A study published in the journal Sleep found that people who sleep fewer than seven hours per night are nearly three times more likely to develop a cold than those who sleep eight hours or more. Quality sleep enhances the body's ability to produce and release cytokines, which help fight off infections and inflammation.

Hormonal Balance and Weight Management: Sleep is crucial for maintaining hormonal balance, particularly those that regulate appetite and metabolism. Poor sleep disrupts the production of ghrelin (which stimulates appetite) and leptin (which signals satiety), leading to increased hunger and cravings for high-calorie foods. A study in the *Annals of Internal Medicine* found that participants who slept only four hours a night had a 28% increase in ghrelin and an 18% decrease in leptin, resulting in weight gain over time.

By understanding the profound impact of sleep on every aspect of our health, it becomes clear why it is essential for longevity. Prioritizing sleep can help reduce the risk of chronic diseases, support cognitive function, boost immunity, and promote hormonal balance, all of which contribute to a longer, healthier life.

Conclusion and Key Takeaways

Sleep is not just a passive state; it is an active, dynamic process critical for maintaining health and promoting longevity. Good sleep supports brain function, cellular repair, immune health, and emotional well-being. It regulates hormones, reduces the risk of chronic diseases, and even helps maintain a healthy weight.

Bonus Content: 10-Day Sleep Improvement Guide

To help you kickstart your journey toward better sleep, here's a simple 10-day sleep improvement guide designed to create lasting habits:

- **Day 1**: Set a consistent bedtime and wake-up time. Aim for 7-9 hours of sleep.
- **Day 2:** Eliminate caffeine after 2 p.m. Replace with herbal teas like chamomile.
- **Day 3:** Create a bedtime routine: read a book, practice deep breathing, or do light stretches.
- **Day 4:** Make your bedroom a sleep sanctuary: dim lights, lower the temperature, and reduce noise.
- **Day 5:** Avoid screens (phones, tablets, computers) for at least one hour before bed.
- **Day 6:** Engage in physical activity during the day but avoid vigorous exercise in the evening.
- **Day 7:** Incorporate a relaxation technique, such as meditation or progressive muscle relaxation.

- **Day 8**: Limit naps to 20-30 minutes and avoid napping late in the afternoon.
- **Day 9:** Eat a light dinner at least 2-3 hours before bedtime to prevent indigestion.
- **Day 10:** Reflect on your progress: How have these changes impacted your sleep? Set long-term goals to maintain these habits.

By following this 10-day guide, you'll build a foundation for better sleep hygiene that supports a healthier, longer life. Sleep is not just an afterthought—it is the key to unlocking your full potential for longevity and well-being.

Chapter 5: Emotional Wellness – The Mind's Role in Living Longer

Introduction: The Power of Emotional Wellness

A few years ago, I met Linda, a woman in her 80s who radiated joy and energy. She wasn't without her share of life's challenges—loss, health issues, and other difficulties—but what struck me was her unwavering optimism. When I asked her secret, she simply smiled and said, "It's all about finding something to be grateful for every day." Linda's story is more than just a feel-good anecdote; it's a testament to the power of emotional wellness.

Research shows that our emotional state directly impacts our physical health and longevity. A study from Harvard University found that people who reported higher levels of life satisfaction and emotional well-being lived longer, healthier lives than those who didn't. Similarly, a groundbreaking study in the Journal of Psychosomatic Research revealed that chronic stress and negative emotions could shorten lifespan by up to 10 years.

Emotional wellness isn't just about feeling good; it's about cultivating a state of mind that supports your physical health and enhances your quality of life. In this chapter, we'll explore how emotions affect our bodies, practical ways to foster a positive mindset, and the importance of building meaningful social connections.

Section 1: Understanding the Mind-Body Connection

The connection between our mind and body is profound and intricate. Our emotions have a direct impact on our physical health, influencing everything from our immune response to our risk of chronic diseases. Here's how:

Stress and Its Impact on Health: Stress is often referred to as the "silent killer" because of its insidious impact on health. When you're stressed, your body releases stress hormones like cortisol and adrenaline, triggering the "fight or flight" response. While this response can be beneficial in short bursts, chronic stress can have a damaging effect. Studies published in Psychological Science show that prolonged exposure to these hormones can lead to increased inflammation, a weakened immune system, and an elevated risk of heart disease, diabetes, and even cancer. Chronic stress has also been linked to shorter telomeres—the protective caps at the ends of chromosomes—accelerating the aging process at a cellular level.

Happiness and Longevity: On the flip side, positive emotions like happiness, joy, and contentment have been shown to enhance health and extend lifespan. A study conducted by the *University College London* found that people who reported higher levels of happiness had a 35% lower risk of dying over a five-year period compared to their less happy peers. Positive emotions reduce stress hormones, lower blood pressure, and promote healthier heart function, all contributing to a longer life.

Mental Resilience and Health: Mental resilience, or the ability to adapt and bounce back from adversity, plays a crucial role in maintaining emotional wellness and overall health. A *2022 study from the American Psychological Association* revealed that individuals with high levels of mental resilience had lower rates of cardiovascular disease, hypertension, and depression. Resilient people tend to have healthier coping mechanisms, such as engaging in physical activity, practicing mindfulness, and seeking social support, which help buffer the negative effects of stress.

Understanding the mind-body connection helps us see why emotional wellness is so vital for longevity. Our thoughts and feelings are not just passing experiences; they have a measurable impact on our physical health and can influence how long and how well we live.

Section 2: Practicing Daily Mindfulness and Gratitude

Cultivating a positive emotional state is essential for longevity, and practices like mindfulness and gratitude can make a significant difference. Here are some practical exercises to help you build these habits:

Mindfulness Meditation: Mindfulness is the practice of being present in the moment, fully engaged with whatever you're doing. Research published in the *Journal of the American Medical Association* has shown that mindfulness meditation can reduce symptoms of anxiety, depression, and chronic pain, all of which can negatively impact longevity. Here's a simple mindfulness exercise to try:

- Find a quiet place to sit comfortably.
- Close your eyes and focus on your breath. Notice the sensation of the air entering and leaving your nostrils.
- If your mind wanders, gently bring your focus back to your breathing.
- Start with five minutes a day and gradually increase the duration as you become more comfortable with the practice.

Gratitude Journaling: Gratitude is the practice of acknowledging and appreciating the positive aspects of your life. Numerous studies, including one from the *University of California, Davis*, have shown that people who regularly practice gratitude report better physical health, lower levels of stress, and greater overall well-being. Try this simple gratitude exercise:

- At the end of each day, write down three things you are grateful for. These could be as simple as a warm cup of coffee, a smile from a stranger, or a supportive friend.
- Reflect on each item and notice how it makes you feel. Let yourself fully experience the positive emotions associated with gratitude.

Loving-Kindness Meditation: This type of meditation focuses on cultivating feelings of compassion and kindness towards yourself and others. According to a study published in *Psychological Bulletin*, loving-kindness meditation has been linked to increased positive emotions, greater life satisfaction, and reduced symptoms of anxiety and depression.

Here's how to practice:
- Sit quietly and close your eyes. Take a few deep breaths to center yourself.
- Repeat phrases like, "May I be happy. May I be healthy. May I be safe. May I live with ease."
- Gradually extend these wishes to others, starting with loved ones and eventually including neutral people and even those with whom you have conflicts.
- Practice this meditation for 10-15 minutes daily to foster a sense of compassion and emotional well-being.

Progressive Muscle Relaxation (PMR): PMR is a technique that involves tensing and relaxing different muscle groups to reduce physical tension and promote relaxation. Research in the Journal of Behavioral Medicine suggests that PMR can lower blood pressure, reduce anxiety, and improve sleep quality, all contributing to better overall health.

To practice PMR:
- Find a quiet, comfortable place to sit or lie down.
- Starting from your toes, tense each muscle group for 5-10 seconds, then release and relax for 20-30 seconds. Move up through your body—feet, calves, thighs, abdomen, arms, neck, and face.
- Focus on the sensation of relaxation and notice any reduction in stress or tension.

By incorporating these practices into your daily routine, you can cultivate a positive emotional state that supports longevity and overall well-being.

Section 3: Building Strong Relationships

Human beings are inherently social creatures, and our relationships significantly impact our health and longevity. Here's how social connections enhance longevity and tips for building and maintaining them:

The Longevity Benefits of Social Connections: Research consistently shows that people with strong social ties live longer, healthier lives. A meta-analysis published in *PLoS Medicine* found that social isolation is as significant a risk factor for early mortality as smoking 15 cigarettes a day. Social connections provide emotional support, reduce stress, and promote healthy behaviors, all of which contribute to better health outcomes.

For example, studies from the *Blue Zones*—areas where people live the longest—reveal that strong social networks and a sense of belonging are common factors among centenarians. These individuals regularly engage with family, friends, and community members, reinforcing a support system that nurtures both emotional and physical health.

Tips for Building and Maintaining Relationships:

- **Stay Connected with Family and Friends:** Make it a priority to regularly communicate with loved ones, whether through phone calls, video chats, or in-person visits. Plan regular activities or outings to foster deeper connections.
- **Join a Group or Club:** Participate in social groups, such as book clubs, sports teams, volunteer organizations, or hobby groups, to meet new people with shared interests. A study from Harvard Health indicates that people who engage in regular group activities have a lower risk of cognitive decline and better mental health.
- **Practice Active Listening:** When interacting with others, focus on truly listening and being present. Show empathy, ask questions, and validate their feelings. This builds trust and strengthens bonds.
- **Give Back to Your Community:** Volunteering or helping others can enhance your sense of purpose and provide opportunities to connect with like-minded individuals. According to research from the Journal of Gerontology, people who engage in volunteer activities have a 24% lower risk of early death than those who do not.
- **Nurture Existing Relationships:** Invest time and energy in nurturing your current relationships. Reach out regularly, express appreciation, and offer support when needed. Healthy relationships are built on mutual respect, understanding, and communication.

Strong social connections provide emotional support, reduce stress, and foster a sense of belonging—all of which are vital for a long, healthy life.

Conclusion and Key Takeaways

Emotional wellness is a cornerstone of longevity. The mind and body are interconnected, and our emotional state profoundly affects our physical health. By managing stress, cultivating positive emotions, and maintaining strong social connections, we can enhance both the quality and length of our lives.

To support emotional wellness, practice mindfulness and gratitude regularly, engage in activities that bring joy and fulfillment, and build meaningful relationships with others. Remember, the journey to emotional wellness isn't about perfection; it's about small, consistent efforts that add up over time.

Prioritize emotional health as much as physical health, and you'll find that a balanced, fulfilled life naturally contributes to longevity.

Bonus Content: Gratitude Journal Template

To help you start a daily gratitude practice, here's a simple template to use:

Daily Gratitude Journal Template

Date: _____

Three Things I'm Grateful For Today:

_____

_____

_____

(Reflect on simple pleasures, meaningful moments, or positive experiences that you are thankful for today. They could be as small as a delicious meal or as significant as reconnecting with a friend.)

One Positive Experience from Today:
- Describe a positive experience you had today. How did it make you feel? Why was it meaningful to you?

A Challenge I Overcame:
- Reflect on a challenge or difficulty you faced today. How did you handle it? What did you learn from the experience?

An Act of Kindness I Witnessed or Performed:
- Write about an act of kindness you either witnessed or performed today. How did it make you feel? What impact did it have on you or others?

Something I'm Looking Forward to Tomorrow:
- Identify something positive or exciting that you're looking forward to tomorrow. It could be a task, event, or personal time you plan to enjoy.

By consistently practicing gratitude with this template, you can foster a more positive mindset, reduce stress, and enhance your emotional well-being, all of which contribute to a longer, healthier life.

Chapter 6: Your Personalized Longevity Plan – Putting It All Together

Introduction: Take Charge of Your Health

Imagine yourself a decade from now—feeling vibrant, energetic, and more alive than ever. What choices have led you there? The truth is, the key to living a longer, healthier life doesn't lie in quick fixes or fads; it's in the small, consistent actions you take every day. Throughout this book, we've explored various aspects of longevity: nutrition, movement, sleep, emotional wellness, and social connections. Now, it's time to put all these elements together into a personalized longevity plan tailored specifically to you.

Taking charge of your health is an empowering journey. It's about making deliberate choices that align with your goals and values. This chapter will guide you in building a customized plan that fits your lifestyle, priorities, and aspirations. Remember, it's not about perfection but about progress. Small, sustainable changes can make a significant impact over time. Let's start creating your path to a longer, healthier life.

Section 1: Building Your Longevity Plan

Creating a personalized longevity plan involves understanding your current lifestyle, identifying areas for improvement, and setting achievable goals. Here's a step-by-step approach to help you design a plan that works for you:

Assess Your Current Lifestyle: Start by taking an honest look at your current habits and routines. Reflect on the following areas:

- **Nutrition:** Are you consuming a balanced diet rich in plant-based foods, healthy fats, and lean proteins? Are there opportunities to reduce processed foods or sugar intake?

- **Physical Activity:** How often do you move your body? Are you incorporating a mix of aerobic, strength, and flexibility exercises?

- **Sleep:** Are you getting 7-9 hours of quality sleep each night? Do you have a consistent bedtime routine?

- **Emotional Wellness:** How do you manage stress? Do you practice mindfulness or gratitude? Are you maintaining strong social connections?

- **Social Connections:** Do you engage with friends, family, or community groups regularly? Do you feel a sense of belonging and support in your relationships?

Use this assessment to pinpoint areas where you're doing well and identify areas that need more attention.

Set SMART Goals: Once you have assessed your current habits, set SMART (Specific, Measurable, Achievable, Relevant, Time-bound) goals to guide your efforts. For example:

- **Specific:** "I will walk for 30 minutes every morning."
- **Measurable:** "I will track my steps using a pedometer or smartphone app."
- **Achievable:** "I will start with a 10-minute walk and gradually increase to 30 minutes over four weeks."
- **Relevant:** "Walking regularly will help me improve my cardiovascular health and mood."
- **Time-bound:** "I will achieve this goal within one month."

Setting clear, realistic goals will help you stay focused and motivated.

Setting clear, realistic goals will help you stay focused and motivated.

Create a Daily Routine: Integrate your goals into your daily schedule. For example, if improving sleep is a priority, establish a consistent bedtime routine that includes winding down activities like reading or meditation. If physical activity is a focus, schedule a specific time each day for exercise. Write down your routine and place it somewhere visible, like on your fridge or in your planner, to remind yourself of your commitments.

Incorporate Micro-Habits: Micro-habits are small, easily achievable actions that, when repeated consistently, lead to significant changes over time. For example:

- **Nutrition:** Start by adding one serving of vegetables to each meal or replacing one sugary drink with water.
- **Movement**: Begin with a 5-minute stretch routine each morning or take the stairs instead of the elevator.
- **Sleep:** Dim the lights an hour before bed or practice a 5-minute relaxation exercise.
- **Emotional Wellness:** Write down one thing you're grateful for each day or spend 5 minutes in mindful breathing.

These micro-habits may seem small, but they are the building blocks of lasting change.

Track Your Progress: Monitoring your progress helps you stay accountable and motivated. Use a journal, app, or spreadsheet to track your habits and reflect on your journey. Celebrate small wins, and recognize that setbacks are a normal part of the process. Reflect on what worked, what didn't, and adjust your plan as needed.

Adjust and Evolve Your Plan: A personalized longevity plan is not set in stone. It should evolve as you do. Regularly review your goals and progress. Are there new areas you want to focus on? Have your priorities changed? Make adjustments to keep your plan aligned with your current needs and aspirations.

Find Your "Why": Understanding why you want to live a longer, healthier life can provide the motivation needed to stick with your plan. Is it to spend more time with loved ones? To feel more energetic and vibrant? To achieve a personal goal? Write down your "why" and refer to it whenever you need a boost of motivation.

Seek Support: Don't go it alone. Share your goals with a friend, family member, or health professional who can offer support and encouragement. Consider joining a community or group with similar goals to foster a sense of accountability and camaraderie.

By following these steps, you'll create a longevity plan tailored to your unique needs and goals, setting yourself up for a healthier, more vibrant future.

Section 2: Habit Formation Techniques

Building new habits can be challenging, but with the right strategies, it's entirely possible. Here are proven techniques to help you establish and maintain healthy habits:

The Two-Minute Rule: Start with habits that take no more than two minutes to complete. This concept, popularized in *Atomic Habits* by James Clear, is about making the first step so easy that you can't say no. For example, if you want to start meditating, begin with just two minutes a day. Once the habit is established, gradually increase the time.

Habit Stacking: Link a new habit to an existing one. In *Tiny Habits* by BJ Fogg, this technique is called "anchoring." Identify a habit you already do daily (like brushing your teeth) and stack a new habit onto it. For instance, "After I brush my teeth, I will spend two minutes stretching." This approach leverages the existing neural pathways of established habits to make adopting new ones easier.

Make it Enjoyable: Combine habits you need to do with activities you enjoy. For instance, listen to your favorite podcast while going for a walk or watch a favorite TV show while doing a stretching routine. Research shows that when we associate positive emotions with a habit, we're more likely to repeat it.

Use Visual Cues: Place reminders in your environment that trigger the desired habit. For example, keep a water bottle on your desk to remind you to stay hydrated or place your workout clothes by your bed to encourage morning exercise. Visual cues make it easier to remember and act on your new habits.

Track Your Habits: Use a habit tracker to monitor your progress. Seeing a visual representation of your streak (such as a calendar or app that tracks daily actions) can be highly motivating. It also helps you recognize patterns and identify areas where you might need extra focus.

Reward Yourself: Reinforce positive habits with rewards. When you achieve a milestone, celebrate it. Treat yourself to something you enjoy, like a relaxing bath, a new book, or a special outing. Rewards create a positive feedback loop that makes the habit more enjoyable and likely to stick.

Accountability Partners: Share your goals with a friend or join a group with similar aspirations. Having someone to check in with or work alongside provides social support and accountability. According to a study in the *Journal of Consulting and Clinical Psychology*, people who have accountability partners are significantly more likely to achieve their goals.

Embrace Imperfection: Understand that building new habits is not about being perfect. There will be days when you fall short or face setbacks, and that's okay. Focus on consistency over perfection. Missing one day doesn't mean you've failed; it's the long-term pattern that matters. Be kind to yourself and keep moving forward.

Reframe Your Mindset: Shift from an "all-or-nothing" mindset to a "progress over perfection" mentality. Recognize that every small step forward is progress. Celebrate the small wins and remind yourself that every effort counts toward your longevity.

By applying these habit formation techniques, you can create sustainable routines that support your health and longevity goals.

Conclusion and Key Takeaways

Your journey to a longer, healthier life starts with a personalized plan that reflects your unique goals, values, and lifestyle. It's not about adopting a rigid regimen but about making small, meaningful changes that you can maintain over time. By setting SMART goals, incorporating micro-habits, and using proven techniques for habit formation, you're setting yourself up for success.

Remember, the key to longevity is consistency. Small, daily actions add up to big results over time. Stay focused on your "why," celebrate your progress, and be gentle with yourself when things don't go as planned. This is a lifelong journey, not a sprint, and every step you take brings you closer to a healthier, more vibrant future.

Bonus Content: 30-Day Longevity Challenge

To help you commit to your new longevity plan, here's a 30-day challenge designed to guide you through small, sustainable changes:

- Week 1: Movement and Hydration
    - **Day 1-3:** Walk for 10-15 minutes
    - **Bonus Content: 30-Day Longevity Challenge**

To help you commit to your new longevity plan, here's a 30-day challenge designed to guide you through small, sustainable changes that build up to a healthier lifestyle:

Week 1: Movement and Hydration
- **Day 1-3**: Walk for 10-15 minutes each day, focusing on maintaining a brisk pace. Carry a water bottle with you to stay hydrated.
- **Day 4-5**: Add a 5-minute stretching routine after your walk, focusing on major muscle groups.
- **Day 6**: Integrate a new type of movement, such as cycling or dancing, for 15 minutes.
- **Day 7:** Rest or engage in light activity, such as a leisurely stroll or gentle yoga.

Week 2: Nutrition and Mindfulness
- **Day 8-9:** Incorporate an extra serving of vegetables into each meal.
- **Day 10-11:** Practice 5 minutes of mindful eating during one meal—focus on chewing slowly and savoring each bite.
- **Day 12**: Replace one sugary drink with water or herbal tea.
- **Day 13-14**: Try a new healthy recipe using plant-based ingredients and share the meal with a friend or family member.

Week 3: Sleep and Emotional Wellness
- **Day 15-16:** Set a consistent bedtime and wake-up time to establish a sleep routine.
- **Day 17:** Dim lights and turn off screens at least one hour before bedtime.
- **Day 18-19:** Practice a 5-minute gratitude exercise before bed, writing down three things you're grateful for.
- **Day 20-21:** Engage in a relaxation technique like deep breathing or meditation for 10 minutes.

Week 4: Social Connections and Reflection

- **Day 22:** Call or visit a friend or family member to strengthen social bonds.
- **Day 23-24:** Participate in a community event or group activity that interests you.
- **Day 25:** Reflect on your progress and identify areas for further improvement.
- **Day 26-27:** Continue practicing a gratitude exercise and add a positive affirmation each morning.
- **Day 28:** Try a new activity, such as a different workout class or a hobby that interests you.
- **Day 29:** Spend time in nature or a quiet place, reflecting on your journey and setting intentions for the future.
- **Day 30:** Celebrate your progress with a small reward and set new goals to continue your longevity journey.

This challenge aims to help you incorporate holistic changes to improve your overall well-being. Remember, the goal is progress, not perfection. Embrace each day with a commitment to making choices that support your long-term health and vitality.

By following this chapter's guidance, you can create a sustainable plan for longevity tailored to your unique needs and preferences, ensuring a healthier, more vibrant future.

Chapter 7: Sticking with It – Staying Motivated for the Long Haul

Introduction: The Challenges of Staying Motivated

We've all been there—starting out on a new health or wellness journey with excitement and enthusiasm, only to find that the initial motivation begins to wane over time. Whether it's sticking to a new diet, maintaining a regular exercise routine, or practicing mindfulness, the challenge often isn't starting; it's staying consistent in the long term.

Common challenges like hitting a plateau, feeling overwhelmed by setbacks, or simply losing sight of why we started in the first place can make it difficult to maintain momentum. Even the most committed among us will face days where motivation is low, and old habits seem easier than forging new ones. But here's the good news: the key to long-term success isn't about maintaining perfect motivation every day. It's about finding strategies that help you keep moving forward, even when the initial excitement has faded.

In this chapter, we'll explore practical ways to maintain motivation, build a supportive network, and embrace the ripple effect of small, consistent changes. Let's dive in and discover how to stay committed to your longevity journey for the long haul.

Section 1: Maintaining Motivation

Maintaining motivation over time requires strategies that help you overcome inevitable obstacles and celebrate progress along the way. Here are some effective approaches:

Overcoming Plateaus: It's normal to experience plateaus—periods where progress seems to stall. When this happens, it's essential not to lose heart. Instead, view plateaus as an opportunity to reassess your approach. Ask yourself if there's something you could change or improve. For example, if your weight loss has stalled, consider adjusting your diet, trying a new form of exercise, or incorporating strength training to build muscle. Remember that plateaus are often temporary and can be overcome with persistence and flexibility.

Celebrate Small Wins: One of the most effective ways to stay motivated is to celebrate small wins. Research from the *Harvard Business Review* shows that recognizing incremental progress is one of the most powerful motivators. Whether it's hitting a milestone in your exercise routine, sticking to your sleep schedule, or trying a new healthy recipe, take time to acknowledge and celebrate these achievements. Reward yourself with something meaningful—like a relaxing day off, a new book, or a favorite activity. These celebrations reinforce positive behavior and keep you motivated.

Find Inspiration: Regularly seek out sources of inspiration to keep your motivation high. This might include reading books or articles on health and wellness, listening to podcasts, or following social media accounts that focus on longevity and healthy living.

Surround yourself with positive stories and uplifting content that remind you of the benefits of your efforts. Additionally, visualize your long-term goals and how reaching them will positively impact your life.

Reflect on Your "Why": Reconnecting with your "why" can reignite your motivation. Remember why you started your journey to longevity in the first place. Was it to feel more energetic, spend more time with loved ones, or avoid health issues that run in your family? Keep a written reminder of your "why" somewhere visible—like on your bathroom mirror or in your planner. Whenever you feel your motivation slipping, take a moment to reflect on your deeper reasons for pursuing a healthier, longer life.

Mix Things Up: Variety can help keep things fresh and exciting. Try new activities, recipes, or wellness practices to prevent boredom. If you've been walking for exercise, consider adding a dance class or a group cycling session. If your meals feel monotonous, explore new cuisines or cooking techniques. Keeping things varied helps maintain interest and motivation.

Practice Self-Compassion: It's easy to be hard on ourselves when we miss a workout, skip meditation, or indulge in less healthy foods. However, practicing self-compassion—treating yourself with the same kindness and understanding you would offer a friend—can help you stay on track. Studies from the *University of California, Berkeley* show that self-compassion is linked to greater emotional resilience and persistence in achieving goals. Instead of criticizing yourself for a misstep, acknowledge it, learn from it, and move forward.

By implementing these strategies, you can keep your motivation strong, even when faced with challenges, and continue making progress toward your longevity goals.

Section 2: Building a Support System
Having a strong support system is vital for maintaining long-term motivation. Here's why it matters and how to build one:

The Power of Accountability Partners: An accountability partner can make a significant difference in sticking to your goals. Studies in the *Journal of Consulting and Clinical Psychology* found that people with accountability partners were significantly more likely to achieve their goals. An accountability partner can be a friend, family member, or colleague who shares similar goals and can provide encouragement, feedback, and a sense of camaraderie. Make regular check-ins with your partner a part of your routine to discuss progress, celebrate successes, and troubleshoot challenges.

Engage in Community Support: Joining a community or group with similar health and wellness goals can provide a sense of belonging and mutual support. Look for local or online groups focused on activities you enjoy, such as walking clubs, yoga classes, cooking workshops, or meditation groups. Being part of a community fosters motivation by creating a network of like-minded individuals who understand your journey and can offer encouragement and advice.

Seek Professional Guidance: Sometimes, the guidance of a professional can be invaluable. A nutritionist, personal trainer, or therapist can provide personalized support, offer expert advice, and help you navigate challenges. Professionals can also help you set realistic goals, track progress, and adjust your plan as needed.

Leverage Digital Tools and Apps: Technology can be a powerful ally in building a support system. Use health and fitness apps to track your progress, join online communities, and connect with others who share your goals. Many apps offer virtual challenges, group activities, and forums where you can find inspiration and support.

Share Your Journey: Don't be afraid to share your health journey with those around you. Talk to friends, family, or coworkers about your goals and why they're important to you. You might be surprised to find that others are on similar paths or are inspired to start their own journey. Sharing your progress and challenges with loved ones can help you feel supported and motivated.

Create a Positive Environment: Surround yourself with people who support and encourage your goals. If certain environments or relationships are making it harder for you to stick to your plan, consider making adjustments. This might mean setting boundaries with people who undermine your efforts or spending more time with those who uplift and inspire you.

Building a solid support system can provide the motivation, encouragement, and accountability you need to stay committed to your longevity goals. Remember, you don't have to do it alone—reach out, connect, and build a network that supports your journey.

Section 3: Embracing the Ripple Effect

Small, consistent changes can have a profound impact on overall health. Here's how:

The Compounding Benefits of Small Changes: Think of your health journey as a ripple effect. Just as a single pebble dropped into water creates ripples that expand outward, small, positive changes in your daily routine can lead to significant improvements over time. For example, swapping a sugary snack for a piece of fruit might seem like a minor change, but over weeks and months, it can reduce your overall sugar intake, improve your energy levels, and support weight management.

Behavioral Momentum: Small, achievable goals build momentum and confidence. When you accomplish a small goal, you feel motivated to tackle a slightly bigger one. This concept, known as "behavioral momentum," is well-documented in psychology. Start with something manageable—like taking a 10-minute walk daily—and gradually increase the intensity or duration. The satisfaction of achieving each small goal will propel you forward.

Cumulative Health Benefits: Every small action adds up. Studies published in the *American Journal of Health Promotion* have shown that even modest increases in physical activity or minor improvements in diet can lead to better health outcomes, such as lower blood pressure, improved cholesterol levels, and reduced risk of chronic diseases. The key is consistency—small, healthy habits performed daily can create substantial benefits over time.

Creating a Feedback Loop: Positive changes can create a feedback loop that encourages further healthy behavior. For example, getting more sleep improves mood and energy levels, making it easier to exercise regularly. Regular exercise, in turn, enhances sleep quality and reduces stress. This positive cycle reinforces each behavior, leading to a healthier lifestyle overall.

Focus on the Journey, Not Just the Destination: Recognize that the journey to better health is ongoing. Celebrate the small victories and acknowledge the effort you're putting in, even if you don't see immediate results. Focusing on the process rather than just the outcome makes it easier to stay motivated, enjoy the journey, and embrace the ripple effect of positive changes.

By embracing the ripple effect of small, consistent changes, you'll build a foundation of healthy habits that supports your overall well-being and longevity.

Conclusion and Key Takeaways

Staying motivated on your journey to a longer, healthier life is about more than just willpower. It involves understanding common challenges, employing practical strategies to maintain motivation, and building a strong support network. By focusing on small, consistent changes and recognizing their cumulative impact, you can stay committed to your goals and enjoy the process.

Remember, motivation ebbs and flows. It's normal to face moments of doubt or discouragement. But with the right strategies and support, you can keep pushing forward, celebrating your progress along the way. Every small step you take brings you closer to a healthier, more vibrant future. Keep moving forward towards your ultimate goal.

Chapter 8: The Role of Supplements in Healthy Aging

Introduction: The Role of Supplements in Supporting Longevity

As we age, maintaining optimal health and vitality becomes more challenging. While a balanced diet, regular exercise, and a healthy lifestyle remain the cornerstone of aging well, many people turn to dietary supplements to fill nutritional gaps, enhance health, and potentially extend longevity. But are these supplements really necessary, and how effective are they in promoting a longer, healthier life?

This chapter will explore the potential benefits and risks of using supplements as part of a healthy aging strategy. We will discuss popular supplements like Omega-3 fatty acids, Vitamin D, and CoQ10, and provide evidence-based guidance on their use. However, it's essential to remember that supplements are not a one-size-fits-all solution. The best approach involves informed decisions based on individual needs, health conditions, and professional medical advice.

Section 1: The Potential Benefits of Supplements for Healthy Aging

Omega-3 Fatty Acids:
Omega-3 fatty acids, particularly EPA and DHA, found in fish oil, are known for their anti-inflammatory properties. Studies, such as those published in the *Journal of the American Heart Association*, have shown that Omega-3 supplements can help reduce the risk of cardiovascular disease, lower triglycerides, and may protect against cognitive decline. Additionally, research from The Lancet indicates that higher Omega-3 levels are associated with a lower risk of mortality, particularly from heart disease.

Vitamin D:
Often referred to as the "sunshine vitamin," Vitamin D is crucial for bone health, immune function, and muscle strength. As people age, their skin becomes less efficient at synthesizing Vitamin D from sunlight, and dietary intake might not be sufficient. According to a study in the *Journal of Clinical Endocrinology & Metabolism*, adequate Vitamin D levels can help reduce the risk of osteoporosis, falls, and fractures in older adults. Some evidence also suggests that Vitamin D may play a role in reducing the risk of certain cancers and autoimmune diseases.

Coenzyme Q10 (CoQ10):
CoQ10 is a powerful antioxidant that helps produce energy in cells and is particularly important for heart health. Levels of CoQ10 naturally decrease with age, and certain medications, like statins, can further deplete it.

Research in the *Journal of the American College of Cardiology* has demonstrated that CoQ10 supplementation can improve symptoms of heart failure, enhance exercise performance, and reduce oxidative stress, which is linked to aging and various diseases.

Magnesium:

Magnesium is vital for many bodily functions, including muscle function, nerve transmission, blood sugar regulation, and bone health. Studies, such as those in the *American Journal of Clinical Nutrition,* suggest that many older adults are deficient in magnesium, which can contribute to conditions like hypertension, heart disease, and osteoporosis. Supplementation may help support cardiovascular health, reduce the risk of Type 2 diabetes, and promote better sleep quality.

Probiotics:

The gut microbiome plays a crucial role in overall health, and maintaining a balanced gut flora is particularly important as we age. Probiotics, beneficial bacteria found in supplements and fermented foods, can help improve digestive health, support the immune system, and may even influence mood and cognitive function. Research from the *Frontiers in Immunology* journal has shown that probiotics can reduce inflammation, enhance immune response, and improve gut health, which is often compromised in older adults.

Curcumin:
Curcumin, the active compound found in turmeric, has potent anti-inflammatory and antioxidant properties. It is being studied for its potential role in preventing age-related diseases like Alzheimer's, arthritis, and heart disease. According to research in the *Journal of the American Chemical Society,* curcumin may reduce inflammation, improve brain function, and lower the risk of neurodegenerative diseases.

Section 2: The Risks and Considerations of Using Supplements

While supplements can offer various health benefits, they also come with potential risks. It is important to approach supplementation carefully and with guidance from healthcare professionals.

Over-supplementation Risks:
Taking high doses of certain vitamins and minerals can be harmful. For example, excessive Vitamin D can lead to hypercalcemia, which can cause nausea, weakness, and kidney problems. High doses of Vitamin E have been linked to an increased risk of hemorrhagic stroke. It is crucial to avoid exceeding the recommended daily allowances unless advised by a healthcare provider.

Interactions with Medications:
Some supplements can interact with prescription medications, potentially diminishing their effectiveness or causing adverse effects. For instance, Omega-3

supplements can increase bleeding risk when taken with blood-thinning medications like warfarin. CoQ10 may reduce the effectiveness of certain chemotherapy drugs. Always consult with a healthcare provider to check for possible interactions.

Quality and Purity Concerns:
Supplements are not as strictly regulated as prescription medications, which can lead to variations in quality and purity. The *Journal of the American Medical Association* has reported cases where supplements contained less active ingredient than stated or were contaminated with harmful substances. Choosing reputable brands that adhere to good manufacturing practices (GMP) and third-party testing can help mitigate these risks.

Individual Needs Vary:
Not everyone needs the same supplements. Factors such as age, gender, diet, pre-existing health conditions, and genetic predispositions play a role in determining what supplements may be beneficial or necessary. For instance, a person with a balanced diet rich in leafy greens may not need extra magnesium, while someone with limited sun exposure might require Vitamin D supplementation.

The Importance of a Whole-Foods Diet:
Supplements are meant to complement, not replace, a healthy diet. Nutrients are best absorbed from whole foods, which provide a complex mix of vitamins, minerals, fiber, and other beneficial compounds. The goal should

always be to obtain as many nutrients as possible from a varied and balanced diet, using supplements only when needed to fill specific gaps.

Section 3: Evidence-Based Guidance on Supplement Use

Consult Healthcare Professionals:
Before starting any new supplement regimen, it is essential to consult with a healthcare provider, such as a doctor or registered dietitian. They can help determine which supplements are appropriate based on individual health needs, potential interactions, and current medications.

Follow Recommended Dosages:
Stick to the recommended dosages provided on the supplement label or by a healthcare provider. Taking more is not necessarily better and can lead to adverse effects.

Choose Quality Products:
Look for supplements that have been tested by third-party organizations, such as the U.S. Pharmacopeia (USP), NSF International, or Consumer Lab. These certifications help ensure that the products meet quality standards and contain the ingredients listed on the label.

Monitor for Side Effects:
Pay attention to how your body responds to new supplements. If you experience any unusual symptoms, such as digestive issues, allergic reactions, or changes in mood, consult your healthcare provider.

Stay Informed:
The field of nutrition and supplements is constantly evolving, with new research emerging regularly. Stay informed by reading reputable sources, such as medical journals or trusted health websites, and discuss any questions or concerns with your healthcare provider.

Conclusion and Key Takeaways

While supplements can play a role in supporting healthy aging, they are not a magic bullet. They should be used thoughtfully and as part of a broader strategy that includes a balanced diet, regular exercise, good sleep, and emotional wellness. Always prioritize whole foods and consult with healthcare professionals before starting any new supplement regimen. Remember, the goal is to enhance your quality of life safely and effectively.

Chapter 9: The Impact of Technology on Longevity

Introduction: Embracing Technology for Healthy Aging

In the modern era, technology is reshaping every aspect of our lives, including how we manage our health and well-being. From wearable fitness trackers that monitor daily activity to telemedicine platforms that offer healthcare consultations from the comfort of our homes, technology is playing an increasingly vital role in promoting healthy aging. It offers innovative tools and resources that can help us stay active, informed, and connected, ultimately contributing to a longer, healthier life.

However, while technology brings many benefits, it also has its downsides, such as increased screen time and the impact of social media on mental health. This chapter will explore how to leverage technology effectively to support longevity, highlighting the best tools, apps, and devices available today, while also discussing strategies to avoid potential pitfalls.

Section 1: How Modern Technology Aids in Healthy Aging

Wearable Fitness Trackers and Health Monitors:
Devices like Fitbit, Apple Watch, and Garmin are popular wearable fitness trackers that help monitor various health metrics, such as steps, heart rate, sleep patterns, and calories burned. According to a study in the *Journal of*

Medical Internet Research, these devices can encourage physical activity by providing real-time feedback, goal-setting, and social support through community features. Many wearables also offer advanced health monitoring features, such as ECG readings and blood oxygen level measurements, which can help detect potential health issues early.

Telemedicine and Remote Health Consultations:
Telemedicine has become a game-changer in healthcare, especially for older adults or those with mobility challenges. Platforms like Teladoc, Amwell, and Doctor on Demand allow patients to consult with healthcare providers remotely, reducing the need for in-person visits. According to research published in the *Journal of the American Medical Association (JAMA)*, telemedicine increases access to care, improves patient outcomes, and reduces healthcare costs by offering timely, convenient medical consultations and follow-ups.

Apps for Health Monitoring and Management:
Numerous apps are available to help monitor and manage various health aspects, from nutrition and hydration to medication adherence. For example, MyFitnessPal tracks dietary intake and helps users set and achieve nutritional goals, while apps like Medisafe offer reminders to take medications on schedule. Studies in *JMIR mHealth and uHealth* have found that such apps can significantly improve adherence to health routines and encourage healthier behaviors by providing easy-to-use tools and personalized feedback.

Virtual Fitness Classes and Online Communities:
 Virtual fitness platforms like Peloton, Daily Burn, and Yoga with Adriene have made it easier for people of all ages to stay active from the comfort of their homes. These platforms offer a wide range of exercise classes, from high-intensity interval training (HIIT) to gentle yoga, catering to different fitness levels and preferences. Additionally, many virtual fitness programs provide social features that allow users to connect, share progress, and support each other, fostering a sense of community and accountability. Research published in the *Journal of Sports Science & Medicine* suggests that online communities can enhance motivation and commitment to regular physical activity.

Digital Tools for Mental Health and Cognitive Function:
 Digital tools and apps can also support mental health and cognitive function. Meditation and mindfulness apps like Headspace, Calm, and Insight Timer offer guided practices to reduce stress and anxiety. Cognitive training apps such as Lumosity and Elevate use games and exercises designed to improve memory, attention, and problem-solving skills. According to a study in the *Journal of Aging and Health*, engaging regularly with these apps can help reduce cognitive decline and support mental well-being in older adults.

Smart Home Devices for Safety and Convenience:
 Smart home devices, such as Amazon Alexa or Google Home, can assist with daily activities, reminders, and emergency response. These devices can be programmed to

remind users to take their medications, turn off appliances, or contact emergency services if needed. Research from the Gerontologist journal indicates that smart home technology can enhance the safety, independence, and quality of life of older adults by providing assistance with routine tasks and emergency alerts.

Section 2: Considerations and Potential Downsides of Technology

While technology offers many benefits for healthy aging, there are also potential downsides that should be considered:

Increased Screen Time:
Prolonged screen time, whether from smartphones, tablets, or computers, can negatively affect physical health, causing eye strain, poor posture, and reduced physical activity. Additionally, excessive screen time is linked to poor sleep quality, particularly when screens are used before bedtime. The *National Sleep Foundation* recommends reducing screen exposure in the evening and using blue light filters to mitigate these effects.

Social Media and Mental Health:
While social media can provide opportunities for connection, it also has potential risks, particularly for mental health. Research published in the *American Journal of Health Behavior* suggests that excessive social media use is associated with increased anxiety, depression, and

feelings of loneliness, especially among older adults who may be less familiar with navigating these platforms. To mitigate these risks, it's important to use social media mindfully, limit time spent online, and focus on positive, supportive communities.

Data Privacy and Security Concerns:
Many digital health tools and apps collect personal health information, which can pose privacy and security risks. According to a report by the *Pew Research Center*, older adults are particularly vulnerable to data breaches and scams. To protect personal information, users should choose reputable apps with strong privacy policies, use complex passwords, and enable two-factor authentication whenever possible.

Over-reliance on Technology:
Relying too heavily on technology for health monitoring or management may inadvertently reduce personal agency and self-awareness. For example, constantly tracking every step or calorie can lead to obsessive behaviors, which can detract from the overall enjoyment of healthy activities. A balanced approach is key—using technology as a tool to support health without becoming overly dependent on it.

Digital Divide and Accessibility Issues:
Not everyone has equal access to technology or feels comfortable using it. Older adults, in particular, may face challenges due to lack of digital literacy or access to devices and reliable internet. Bridging the digital divide is

crucial for ensuring that all individuals, regardless of age or background, can benefit from technological advances in healthcare. Community programs and resources that provide digital education and support can help address these disparities.

Section 3: Strategies for Using Technology Mindfully

Set Time Limits:

Establish boundaries for screen time, particularly for non-essential activities like social media. Use features like screen time monitors or app usage trackers to help manage digital consumption.

Prioritize In-Person Interactions:

While technology can help maintain connections, prioritize face-to-face interactions whenever possible. In-person contact has been shown to provide stronger social and emotional benefits than digital communication alone.

Choose High-Quality Tools:

Research and select apps and devices that have strong user reviews, data privacy measures, and evidence-based benefits. Seek out platforms that offer genuine health benefits and avoid those that seem gimmicky or overly commercial.

Practice Digital Mindfulness:
Incorporate mindfulness techniques when using digital tools. Take regular breaks, practice deep breathing, or use apps specifically designed for mindfulness and relaxation.

Educate and Stay Informed:
Stay informed about potential privacy risks and best practices for online security. Regularly update passwords, review privacy settings, and stay aware of the latest digital scams or vulnerabilities.

Balance Tech Use with Offline Activities:
Make time for non-digital activities that promote well-being, such as spending time in nature, reading a physical book, or engaging in hobbies that don't require screens.

Conclusion and Key Takeaways

Technology offers numerous tools and resources that can aid in healthy aging, from wearable fitness trackers and telemedicine to digital tools for mental health and cognitive function. However, it's essential to use technology mindfully and balance it with offline activities to avoid potential downsides, such as increased screen time or negative mental health effects. By leveraging technology wisely, we can harness its potential to support longevity and overall well-being.

Chapter 10: Stress Management for Longevity

Introduction: The Importance of Managing Stress for Longevity

Stress is an inevitable part of life, but how we manage it can significantly impact our health and longevity. Chronic stress has been linked to numerous health issues, including cardiovascular disease, weakened immune function, cognitive decline, and accelerated aging. In today's fast-paced world, managing stress is more critical than ever for maintaining a healthy, balanced life.

This chapter will explore the science behind stress and aging, highlighting how unmanaged stress affects the body over time. We'll delve into various evidence-based techniques for managing stress, such as mindfulness, meditation, breathing exercises, nature therapy, and journaling, and offer practical tips on how to incorporate these practices into daily life for improved well-being and a longer, healthier life.

Section 1: The Science Behind Stress and Aging

How Stress Affects the Body and Mind:
When we encounter a stressful situation, our bodies initiate a "fight or flight" response, releasing stress hormones like cortisol and adrenaline. While these hormones are helpful in short bursts, chronic activation due to ongoing stress can lead to harmful effects on health. According to

research published in the *Journal of the American Medical Association (JAMA)*, chronic stress contributes to inflammation, elevated blood pressure, and higher cholesterol levels, which can increase the risk of heart disease, stroke, and other conditions.

The Impact of Stress on Cellular Aging:
Studies have shown that chronic stress can accelerate aging at the cellular level by shortening telomeres, the protective caps on the ends of chromosomes. Telomeres naturally shorten as we age, but stress can speed up this process, leading to premature cellular aging. Research from the *Proceedings of the National Academy of Sciences (PNAS)* found that people with chronic stress had significantly shorter telomeres than those with lower stress levels, which could translate to a reduced lifespan.

Cognitive Decline and Mental Health:
Chronic stress negatively impacts brain function and mental health. High levels of cortisol can damage the hippocampus, a brain region critical for memory and learning. Over time, this can contribute to cognitive decline and increase the risk of neurodegenerative diseases like Alzheimer's. According to a study published in *Neurology*, individuals with high levels of stress are at a higher risk of developing mild cognitive impairment (MCI) and other forms of dementia.

Immune Function and Disease Susceptibility:
Stress suppresses the immune system, making the body
more susceptible to infections and diseases. Chronic stress
can decrease the body's ability to produce lymphocytes,
the white blood cells that help fight off infections. A study
in the Psychosomatic Medicine journal demonstrated that
individuals with high-stress levels are more likely to catch
colds, flu, and other illnesses due to compromised immune
function.

Section 2: Effective Techniques for Stress Management

Mindfulness Meditation:
Mindfulness meditation involves paying attention to the
present moment without judgment. This practice can
reduce stress by calming the mind and reducing the
overactivity of the sympathetic nervous system. Research
from the American Psychological Association shows that
regular mindfulness practice can lower cortisol levels,
reduce anxiety, and improve emotional regulation.
- **Practice Tip:** Start with 5-10 minutes daily of focusing
  on your breath, a mantra, or your bodily sensations.
  Gradually increase the duration as you become more
  comfortable with the practice.

Breathing Exercises:
Deep breathing exercises can activate the parasympathetic
nervous system, responsible for the "rest and digest"
response, which counteracts the body's stress response.
Techniques such as diaphragmatic breathing, box

breathing, and alternate nostril breathing have been shown to reduce stress and anxiety, as demonstrated in a study published in the Journal of Clinical Psychology.

- **Practice Tip:** Try diaphragmatic breathing by inhaling deeply through your nose, allowing your abdomen to expand, and then exhaling slowly through your mouth. Repeat for 5-10 minutes to promote relaxation.

Nature Therapy (Ecotherapy):

Spending time in nature has been shown to reduce stress, anxiety, and depression while enhancing overall well-being. The practice, often referred to as "forest bathing" or Shinrin-yoku, has roots in Japanese culture and is supported by numerous studies. A meta-analysis in the International Journal of Environmental Research and Public Health found that nature exposure significantly lowers cortisol levels and reduces perceived stress.

- **Practice Tip:** Aim to spend at least 20-30 minutes in nature several times a week. This could be a walk in the park, gardening, or simply sitting outside.

Journaling:

Journaling allows individuals to express and process their thoughts and emotions, which can help manage stress. According to research in the *Journal of Research in Personality*, expressive writing can improve mental well-being, reduce symptoms of anxiety and depression, and enhance emotional regulation.

- **Practice Tip:** Set aside 10-15 minutes daily to write about your thoughts, feelings, and experiences. Focus on gratitude, challenges, and areas for personal growth.

Physical Activity:

Regular physical activity is one of the most effective stress management techniques. Exercise helps release endorphins —natural mood elevators—and reduces levels of stress hormones like cortisol. A study in the *Journal of Health Psychology* found that participants who engaged in regular exercise reported lower stress levels and greater overall well-being.

- **Practice Tip:** Incorporate at least 30 minutes of moderate exercise, such as walking, jogging, dancing, or yoga, into your daily routine.

Progressive Muscle Relaxation (PMR):

PMR involves tensing and relaxing different muscle groups to reduce physical tension and promote relaxation. Studies in the Journal of Behavioral Medicine suggest that PMR can lower blood pressure, reduce anxiety, and improve sleep quality.

- **Practice Tip**: Find a quiet place to sit or lie down. Tense each muscle group for 5-10 seconds, then release and relax for 20-30 seconds, moving from your toes to your head.

Section 3: Practical Guide to Incorporating Stress Management Techniques

Start Small and Be Consistent:
Begin by incorporating one or two stress management techniques into your daily routine. Start with just a few minutes each day and gradually increase the duration or number of practices. Consistency is key to building resilience over time.

Create a Relaxing Environment:
Designate a calm, quiet space in your home for stress management activities like meditation, breathing exercises, or journaling. Use soothing elements like soft lighting, calming scents (lavender or chamomile), or relaxing music to enhance your experience.

Set Reminders and Prioritize Self-Care:
Use reminders on your phone or sticky notes to schedule time for stress management practices. Treat this time as a non-negotiable self-care appointment. Prioritizing self-care is essential for maintaining long-term health and well-being.

Integrate Techniques into Existing Routines:
Incorporate stress management techniques into existing routines. For example, practice deep breathing exercises while waiting in line or mindful walking during your commute. This integration makes it easier to adopt and sustain new habits.

Seek Social Support:
Share your stress management goals with friends, family, or support groups. Having accountability partners can encourage adherence to stress management practices and provide emotional support during challenging times.

Monitor Your Progress:
Keep a journal to track your progress, noting how you feel before and after practicing stress management techniques. Reflect on the benefits you experience and adjust your approach as needed to maintain effectiveness.

Conclusion and Key Takeaways

Managing stress is essential for maintaining health and promoting longevity. By understanding the impact of stress on the body and mind and incorporating proven techniques like mindfulness, meditation, breathing exercises, nature therapy, and journaling into your daily routine, you can build resilience and enhance overall well-being. Remember, small, consistent changes can lead to significant improvements in health over time. Make stress management a priority and take proactive steps to live a longer, healthier life.

Chapter 11: Understanding and Leveraging Genetics for Healthy Aging

Introduction: The Role of Genetics in Aging

Genetics plays a crucial role in determining how we age, influencing everything from our susceptibility to certain diseases to our overall lifespan. However, genetics is not destiny. Research in the field of epigenetics—how lifestyle and environmental factors can influence the expression of our genes—suggests that while we may inherit certain predispositions, our daily choices can significantly impact how these genetic tendencies manifest.

This chapter will explain the role of genetics in aging, explore how lifestyle choices can modify genetic expression, and discuss how to use genetic testing to personalize health and wellness plans. We will also consider the limitations and ethical concerns surrounding genetic testing and provide actionable steps readers can take based on their genetic predispositions to promote healthy aging.

Section 1: Genetics and Aging – The Basics

The Genetic Blueprint of Aging:
Our genetic code, comprised of DNA, contains the instructions for building and maintaining our bodies. Certain genes are directly involved in the aging process, such as those regulating cellular repair, immune function,

and inflammation. For instance, the APOE gene is linked to the risk of developing Alzheimer's disease, while variants in the FOXO3 gene are associated with longevity and enhanced resistance to age-related diseases.

Epigenetics: Beyond the DNA Sequence:
While our genetic code is fixed, epigenetics refers to changes in gene expression that do not involve alterations to the underlying DNA sequence. Epigenetic changes are influenced by environmental factors such as diet, exercise, sleep, stress, and exposure to toxins. For example, research in the *Journal of Gerontology* shows that lifestyle factors like regular physical activity and a healthy diet can positively impact the expression of genes related to aging, reducing the risk of chronic diseases and promoting a longer lifespan.

The Heritability of Longevity:
Studies estimate that genetics account for about 20-30% of an individual's lifespan, while lifestyle and environmental factors make up the rest. According to a study published in *Nature Communications*, people with long-lived parents are more likely to live longer themselves, suggesting a hereditary component. However, lifestyle choices still play a critical role in determining how genetic predispositions manifest.

Gene-Environment Interactions:
The interaction between genes and the environment is complex and bidirectional. For example, while someone may have a genetic predisposition to obesity, regular exercise and a healthy diet can mitigate this risk.

Conversely, a sedentary lifestyle and poor diet can exacerbate genetic susceptibility to certain diseases. Research from the *American Journal of Epidemiology* emphasizes the importance of understanding gene-environment interactions to develop effective personalized health strategies.

Section 2: Using Genetic Testing to Personalize Health and Wellness

What is Genetic Testing?
Genetic testing involves analyzing DNA to identify genetic variations that may influence an individual's health, risk of diseases, and response to certain medications. Tests can range from broad assessments of ancestry and traits (like those offered by 23andMe or AncestryDNA) to more targeted tests that examine specific genes related to health, such as BRCA1 and BRCA2 for breast cancer risk.

How Genetic Testing Can Guide Personalized Health Plans:
Genetic testing can help individuals make more informed decisions about their health by identifying predispositions to certain conditions, such as heart disease, diabetes, or certain cancers. For example, if a genetic test reveals a higher risk for Type 2 diabetes, an individual might prioritize weight management, blood sugar control, and regular physical activity to mitigate that risk.

Additionally, genetic testing can guide personalized nutrition plans, often referred to as "nutrigenomics." Studies in the Journal of Nutrition suggest that certain genetic variations affect how we metabolize nutrients, which can impact our dietary needs. For example, some people may be more sensitive to caffeine or more prone to deficiencies in specific vitamins like B12, guiding tailored dietary recommendations.

Limitations and Ethical Concerns of Genetic Testing:
While genetic testing can provide valuable insights, it also has limitations and ethical concerns:

- **Predictive Uncertainty:** A genetic predisposition does not guarantee the development of a disease; it simply indicates a higher risk. For instance, having a gene variant associated with Alzheimer's does not mean one will definitely develop the condition, as other factors like lifestyle and environment also play a significant role.
- **Privacy and Discrimination:** Genetic information is sensitive, and there are concerns about data privacy and the potential for genetic discrimination by employers or insurers. The Genetic Information Nondiscrimination Act (GINA) in the United States provides some protection, but limitations still exist.
- **Emotional Impact:** Learning about potential health risks can cause anxiety or stress, and not everyone may feel equipped to handle this information. It's essential to seek genetic counseling before and after testing to fully understand the results and implications.

Ethical Considerations and Responsible Use of Genetic Information:

When considering genetic testing, it is crucial to evaluate the potential benefits and drawbacks. Discussing the decision with a healthcare provider or genetic counselor can provide clarity on whether testing is appropriate and how to interpret the results responsibly. Genetic counselors are trained to help individuals understand their genetic risks and the implications of testing, including the psychological and social impact.

Section 3: Actionable Steps Based on Genetic Predispositions

Seek Professional Guidance:

Work with healthcare professionals, including genetic counselors, dietitians, and doctors, to interpret genetic test results and develop a personalized plan. This collaboration can help you understand your risks and the best strategies to mitigate them.

Adopt a Healthy Lifestyle:

Regardless of genetic predispositions, certain lifestyle choices benefit everyone. Regular physical activity, a balanced diet rich in fruits, vegetables, and whole grains, adequate sleep, stress management, and avoiding smoking and excessive alcohol consumption are fundamental to healthy aging. A study published in the British Medical Journal (BMJ) suggests that even individuals with a high genetic risk for heart disease can significantly reduce their risk by adhering to a healthy lifestyle.

Focus on Epigenetic Modifications:
Engage in behaviors that positively influence epigenetic changes. For example:

- **Nutrition:** Consuming a diet high in antioxidants and anti-inflammatory foods can promote healthy gene expression.
- **Physical Activity:** Regular exercise has been shown to positively affect gene expression related to metabolism, inflammation, and overall health.
- **Stress Management:** Practices like mindfulness meditation, yoga, and deep breathing can reduce stress and may influence genes associated with aging and longevity.

Consider Tailored Nutritional and Exercise Plans:
Use genetic information to customize your health approach. For example, if you have a genetic predisposition for low vitamin D levels, you might prioritize vitamin D-rich foods or supplements. If you have a family history of cardiovascular disease, focus on heart-healthy foods and exercises known to improve cardiovascular function.

Regular Monitoring and Reassessment:
Your health plan should be dynamic and adaptable to changes over time. Regularly review your genetic and health information with healthcare professionals to make any necessary adjustments based on new findings or evolving personal health needs.

Educate Yourself About Genetic Research:
Stay informed about new developments in genetics and epigenetics that may impact your health strategies. Research in this field is rapidly evolving, and new studies can provide updated guidance on how best to use genetic information to support healthy aging.

Conclusion and Key Takeaways

While genetics play a role in determining how we age, they do not dictate our fate. Advances in genetic testing offer powerful tools for understanding our predispositions and tailoring personalized health strategies. However, it is essential to approach genetic testing thoughtfully, considering its limitations and ethical concerns. By leveraging genetic information wisely and making informed lifestyle choices, we can optimize our health and longevity.

Personal Stories and Case Studies

Including personal stories or case studies can help bring the concepts in your book to life, making them more relatable and inspiring for readers. Below are a few examples of fictionalized narratives that illustrate how individuals have successfully applied the strategies discussed in your book to improve their health, manage stress, and leverage technology for longevity.

Case Study 1: Lisa's Journey to a Healthier Life Through Mindful Eating and Movement

Lisa, a 52-year-old working professional and mother of two, found herself struggling with low energy, poor sleep, and a creeping sense of discomfort with her weight. Like many, she was caught in a cycle of stress eating and sporadic exercise. After reading about the importance of movement and nutrition for longevity, she decided to make small, manageable changes to her lifestyle.

Lisa began by incorporating more plant-based foods into her diet, as suggested in Chapter 3, "Nutrition for Longevity." She started with one plant-based meal a day and slowly increased the proportion of vegetables and whole grains in her diet. To her surprise, she began to feel more energetic and less bloated. Encouraged by this progress, she decided to add daily movement to her routine. She began with brisk 20-minute walks around her neighborhood and eventually worked up to participating in local dance classes, something she had loved in her younger years.

Within a few months, Lisa noticed improvements in her sleep quality, mood, and overall sense of well-being. Her friends and family also saw the positive changes, and she even inspired a few colleagues to join her in morning walks. Lisa's experience highlights how small, consistent changes can have a powerful ripple effect on overall health and longevity.

Case Study 2: Mark's Stress Management Transformation with Mindfulness and Technology

Mark, 60, had always been a high achiever. He prided himself on his work ethic, but his demanding career had led to chronic stress, poor sleep, and frequent headaches. After his doctor warned him about his elevated blood pressure, Mark realized he needed to find a way to manage his stress more effectively.

He decided to try the mindfulness practices discussed in Chapter 10, "Stress Management for Longevity." Mark downloaded a meditation app, Calm, and started with short, 5-minute guided sessions each morning. Initially skeptical, he quickly found that these brief sessions helped him feel calmer and more centered at the start of each day.

Inspired by his initial success, Mark began incorporating more stress management techniques into his routine.

He practiced deep breathing exercises during his lunch break and took short walks in the nearby park after work to benefit from nature therapy. Mark also set reminders on his smartwatch to pause and practice gratitude, as outlined in Chapter 5, "Emotional Wellness."

After several weeks, Mark noticed a significant reduction in his stress levels. His sleep improved, his headaches became less frequent, and his blood pressure gradually normalized. Mark's journey shows the impact of combining mindfulness, movement, and technology to enhance health and well-being.

Case Study 3: Sarah's Use of Genetic Testing for Personalized Health Planning

At 45, Sarah had always considered herself relatively healthy, but her family history of diabetes and heart disease worried her. She wanted to be proactive about her health but wasn't sure where to start. After reading about the potential of genetic testing in Chapter 11, "Understanding and Leveraging Genetics for Healthy Aging," she decided to take a DNA test to learn more about her specific risks.

The test results indicated that Sarah had a higher-than-average risk for Type 2 diabetes and certain heart conditions. Armed with this knowledge, she consulted with a nutritionist and a genetic counselor to create a personalized health plan. Her plan included a diet tailored to her genetic profile, focusing on reducing sugar and refined carbs while incorporating more whole grains, lean proteins, and healthy fats.

Sarah also began a regular exercise routine that included both cardio and strength training, as suggested in Chapter 2, "The Power of Movement." Within a few months, Sarah had lost weight, felt more energetic, and saw improvements in her blood sugar levels. She continues to monitor her progress with the help of her healthcare team and feels empowered by her ability to make informed choices about her health.

Sarah's story demonstrates how genetic insights, combined with personalized health strategies, can help manage risk and promote longevity.

Case Study 4: James' Embrace of Technology for Heart Health Monitoring

James, a 67-year-old retired engineer, had recently been diagnosed with atrial fibrillation, a condition that increased his risk of stroke. Concerned about his health, James wanted a way to monitor his heart more closely without constant trips to the doctor.

He decided to invest in a smartwatch with a built-in ECG function, as mentioned in Chapter 9, "The Impact of Technology on Longevity." The device allowed him to monitor his heart rhythm regularly and detect any irregularities. The data collected on the watch was shared with his cardiologist, enabling them to adjust his treatment plan proactively.

James also used the watch to track his steps and set daily walking goals. He joined an online community of people with similar health challenges, where he found support, motivation, and practical advice. This technological approach gave him peace of mind, knowing that he could actively participate in managing his condition.

James's story illustrates the role of technology in supporting healthy aging, offering tools to monitor health metrics and create a community of support.

Bonus Content: Long-Term Vision Board Exercise

A vision board is a powerful tool to help you visualize your future self and set long-term goals. By creating a visual representation of your aspirations, you engage your mind in a creative and motivating way that keeps your goals at the forefront of your daily life. Here's a step-by-step guide to creating your vision board:

- **Gather Materials:** Start with a blank canvas, poster board, or digital platform. Gather magazines, newspapers, or printouts of images and words that resonate with your goals and aspirations. You'll also need scissors, glue, markers, and any other creative supplies you like.
- **Reflect on Your Goals:** Take a few moments to reflect on what you want to achieve in the long term. What does a healthy, fulfilling life look like to you? Consider different areas like health, relationships, personal growth, and adventure. Write down your thoughts to clarify your vision.
- **Select Images and Words:** Choose images, words, or phrases that inspire and represent your goals. Look for visuals that evoke positive emotions and align with your desired lifestyle. For example, if you want to improve your fitness, you might choose pictures of people exercising outdoors or engaging in activities you enjoy.
- **Create Your Board:** Arrange your images and words on your board in a way that feels meaningful to you. There's no right or wrong way—this is your personal vision. Be creative and enjoy the process.

Conclusion: The Path to a Longer, Healthier Life

As we reach the end of this book, it's important to remember that the journey to a longer, healthier life is not a destination but an ongoing process. The path to longevity is paved with daily choices—choices about what we eat, how we move, how we manage stress, and how we nurture our minds and bodies.

Throughout these chapters, we've explored the many facets of healthy aging: from understanding the science of longevity and adopting the right daily habits, to leveraging modern tools like technology and genetic testing. We've seen that while genetics play a role, they do not dictate our fate; our lifestyle choices have the power to shape how we age, protect us from disease, and enhance our overall well-being.

The information and strategies shared in this book are not meant to overwhelm you with change but to inspire you to make small, sustainable adjustments that fit into your unique life. Even modest changes, when practiced consistently, can have profound effects over time. The goal is progress, not perfection.

Embrace Your Journey
Every step you take toward healthier habits is a step toward a brighter future. Celebrate your victories, no matter how small, and be kind to yourself on days when things don't go as planned. Remember, it's the cumulative

effect of these choices—day by day, habit by habit—that ultimately shapes your health and longevity. Longevity is not just about adding years to your life; it's about adding life to your years. It's about waking up each day with energy, purpose, and the knowledge that you're doing everything you can to live your best life, for as long as possible.

Looking Ahead

As you move forward, I encourage you to revisit the strategies in this book, experiment with what works best for you, and continue learning. The fields of health, wellness, and longevity are constantly evolving, and new research and insights will continue to emerge. Stay curious, stay informed, and stay committed to your journey.

Above all, remember that every day is an opportunity to make choices that benefit your health, happiness, and longevity. You have the power to shape your future, and I hope this book has given you the tools, knowledge, and inspiration to do just that.

Thank you for taking this journey with me.

With gratitude and best wishes,

Naomi Allen

Frequently Asked Questions (FAQ) Section

FAQ: Starting and Sustaining Healthy Habits
How do I start if I feel overwhelmed?
Start small and focus on one habit at a time. It's easy to feel overwhelmed when making lifestyle changes, especially if you're trying to tackle multiple areas at once. Begin with a simple, manageable step, like adding an extra serving of vegetables to your meals or taking a 10-minute walk each day. Celebrate these small victories, and gradually build on them. Remember, consistency is more important than intensity when forming new habits.

Can I really change my habits later in life?
Absolutely! It's never too late to make positive changes. Research shows that even small modifications in diet, exercise, and other lifestyle factors can have significant health benefits, regardless of age. The brain remains plastic—capable of learning and adapting—throughout our lives. Start with achievable goals, and use techniques like habit stacking (pairing a new habit with an existing one) to help changes stick.

How do I find the right balance between technology use and mindful living?
Use technology as a tool, not a crutch. Technology can support healthy aging by providing access to fitness apps, health monitors, and virtual communities, but it's important to use it mindfully. Set boundaries for screen time, especially before bed, and prioritize in-person

interactions and offline activities. Aim for balance by using technology to enhance, not replace, real-life connections and mindful practices.

What if I have specific health conditions?
Always consult with a healthcare professional before making significant lifestyle changes, especially if you have existing health conditions. This book offers general guidance, but personalized advice from a doctor, dietitian, or other specialists will ensure your approach is safe and effective for your unique situation. Tailor the strategies in the book to suit your individual needs and work with your healthcare provider to monitor your progress.

Is it worth getting genetic testing to personalize my health plan?
Genetic testing can provide valuable insights into your predispositions for certain health conditions, but it's not necessary for everyone. If you have a family history of specific diseases or want to tailor your diet and exercise plan more closely to your genetic profile, testing could be helpful. However, genetics is only one piece of the puzzle. Your lifestyle choices—like diet, exercise, and stress management—still play a critical role in your overall health.

FAQ: Managing Stress and Emotional Wellness
How can I reduce stress in my daily life?
Start by incorporating small stress-reducing practices into your daily routine, like deep breathing exercises, mindfulness meditation, or short nature walks. Identify your stress triggers and develop coping strategies, such as

journaling or talking with a friend. Remember, managing stress is an ongoing process, and finding the right combination of techniques takes time. Regular practice and self-compassion are key.

What are some practical ways to practice mindfulness?
Mindfulness can be practiced in many ways, from meditation to mindful eating or even mindful walking. Begin by paying full attention to the present moment—notice the sights, sounds, smells, and sensations around you. You can also use apps like Calm or Headspace for guided sessions. Start with just a few minutes a day, gradually increasing as you feel more comfortable.

FAQ: Nutrition and Physical Activity
Do I need to follow a specific diet to live longer?
No single diet fits everyone, but focusing on whole, plant-based foods, lean proteins, and healthy fats is a good general guideline. Consider adopting principles from diets that have been associated with longevity, like the Mediterranean or Blue Zone diets, which emphasize fruits, vegetables, whole grains, nuts, and healthy fats like olive oil. Find a diet that works for you, is sustainable, and provides all the nutrients your body needs.

How much exercise is necessary for healthy aging?
Aim for at least 150 minutes of moderate-intensity aerobic activity (like brisk walking) per week, combined with muscle-strengthening activities on two or more days per week.

Flexibility and balance exercises, like yoga or tai chi, are also beneficial, especially as you age. However, it's important to start at a level that is comfortable for you and gradually increase the duration and intensity.

Can supplements really help with healthy aging?
Supplements can play a role in supporting healthy aging, but they should not replace a balanced diet. Some supplements, like Vitamin D, Omega-3 fatty acids, and CoQ10, may be beneficial, especially if you have deficiencies. Always consult with a healthcare provider before starting any new supplement regimen to ensure it's appropriate for your individual needs and does not interact with any medications.

FAQ: Motivation and Long-Term Success
How do I stay motivated when progress feels slow?
Focus on small, measurable goals and celebrate every achievement, no matter how minor it seems. Motivation can wane when progress feels slow, but recognizing and rewarding yourself for sticking with your habits can help maintain momentum. Use tools like a habit tracker, join a community for support, or find an accountability partner to keep you on track.

What if I struggle to keep up with new habits?
It's normal to face challenges when building new habits. Start by assessing why you're struggling—are the changes too ambitious? Are there barriers in your environment?

Break down your goals into even smaller steps, and remember, it's okay to start over. Be kind to yourself and recognize that every attempt is a step toward lasting change.

References:

Chapter 1: Longevity Unveiled – Understanding the Science Behind a Long Life

National Institute on Aging. (2022). What Do We Know About Healthy Aging?

Harvard Health Publishing. (2023). The Biology of Aging: Cellular and Molecular Aspects. Harvard Medical School.

Buettner, D. (2012). The Blue Zones: 9 Lessons for Living Longer From the People Who've Lived the Longest. National Geographic.

Chapter 2: The Power of Movement – How Moving Your Body Fuels Longevity

Warburton, D. E. R., & Bredin, S. S. D. (2017). Health benefits of physical activity: A systematic review of current systematic reviews. Current Opinion in Cardiology, 32(5), 541-556.

Lee, I.-M., Shiroma, E. J., Lobelo, F., Puska, P., Blair, S. N., & Katzmarzyk, P. T. (2012). Effect of physical inactivity on major non-communicable diseases worldwide: An analysis of burden of disease and life expectancy. The Lancet, 380(9838), 219-229.

Harvard T.H. Chan School of Public Health. (2023). Exercise and Physical Activity.

Chapter 3: Nutrition for Longevity – Eating for a Longer Life

Willett, W. C., & Ludwig, D. S. (2011). The US Dietary Guidelines: Scientific Shortcomings. The Lancet, 378(9793), 373-375.

Martínez-González, M. A., & Corella, D. (2014). Mediterranean diet and health: Evidence from observational and intervention studies. British Journal of Nutrition, 111(S2), S30-S35.
National Center for Biotechnology Information (NCBI). (2022). Health benefits of dietary fiber.

Chapter 4: Sleep and Longevity – How Rest Recharges Your Life Span

Walker, M. (2017). Why We Sleep: Unlocking the Power of Sleep and Dreams. Scribner.
National Sleep Foundation. (2023). Sleep and Health.
Cappuccio, F. P., D'Elia, L., Strazzullo, P., & Miller, M. A. (2010). Sleep duration and all-cause mortality: A systematic review and meta-analysis of prospective studies. Sleep, 33(5), 585-592.

Chapter 5: Emotional Wellness – The Mind's Role in Living Longer

Davidson, R. J., & McEwen, B. S. (2012). Social influences on neuroplasticity: Stress and interventions to promote well-being. Nature Neuroscience, 15(5), 689-695.
American Psychological Association. (2023). Mind-Body Health: Stress.
Seligman, M. E. P. (2011). Flourish: A Visionary New Understanding of Happiness and Well-being. Free Press.

Chapter 6: Your Personalized Longevity Plan – Putting It All Together

Clear, J. (2018). *Atomic Habits: An Easy & Proven Way to Build Good Habits & Break Bad Ones.* Avery.

Fogg, B. J. (2019). *Tiny Habits: The Small Changes That Change Everything.* Houghton Mifflin Harcourt.

Duckworth, A. L. (2016). *Grit: The Power of Passion and Perseverance.* Scribner.

Chapter 7: Sticking with It – Staying Motivated for the Long Haul

Baumeister, R. F., & Tierney, J. (2011). *Willpower: Rediscovering the Greatest Human Strength.* Penguin Books.

Heath, C., & Heath, D. (2010). *Switch: How to Change Things When Change Is Hard.* Crown Business.

Duhigg, C. (2012). *The Power of Habit: Why We Do What We Do in Life and Business.* Random House.

Chapter 8: The Role of Supplements in Healthy Aging

Calder, P. C. (2013). Omega-3 polyunsaturated fatty acids and inflammatory processes: Nutrition or pharmacology? *British Journal of Clinical Pharmacology, 75*(3), 645-662.

Holick, M. F. (2007). Vitamin D deficiency. *New England Journal of Medicine, 357*(3), 266-281.

Gorton, H. C., & Jarvis, K. (1999). The effectiveness of vitamin C in preventing and relieving the symptoms of virus-induced respiratory infections. *Journal of Manipulative and Physiological Therapeutics, 22*(8), 530-533.

Chapter 9: The Impact of Technology on Longevity

Loria, K. (2018). How fitness trackers can help you meet your health goals — or get in your way. Business Insider.

Bashshur, R., Shannon, G., Krupinski, E., & Grigsby, J. (2013). The empirical foundations of telemedicine interventions for chronic disease management. Telemedicine and e-Health, 19(10), 744-787.

Bratman, G. N., Hamilton, J. P., & Daily, G. C. (2012). The impacts of nature experience on human cognitive function and mental health. Annals of the New York Academy of Sciences, 1249(1), 118-136.

Chapter 10: Stress Management for Longevity

Sapolsky, R. M. (2004). Why Zebras Don't Get Ulcers: The Acclaimed Guide to Stress, Stress-Related Diseases, and Coping. Holt Paperbacks.

Kabat-Zinn, J. (2003). Mindfulness-Based Interventions in Context: Past, Present, and Future. Clinical Psychology: Science and Practice, 10(2), 144-156.

Packer, M. (2021). Breathing Exercises and Mindfulness Meditation for Mental Health and Cognitive Function. Journal of Alternative and Complementary Medicine, 27(3), 195-202.

Chapter 11: Understanding and Leveraging Genetics for Healthy Aging

Christensen, K., Johnson, T. E., & Vaupel, J. W. (2006). The quest for genetic determinants of human longevity: Challenges and insights. Nature Reviews Genetics, 7(6), 436-448.

Loomba, R., & Sanyal, A. J. (2013). The global NAFLD epidemic. Nature Reviews Gastroenterology & Hepatology, 10(11), 686-690.

Feinberg, A. P. (2018). The Key Role of Epigenetics in Human Disease Prevention and Mitigation. New England Journal of Medicine, 378(6), 1323-1334. Link

Collins, F. S., & Varmus, H. (2015). A New Initiative on Precision Medicine. New England Journal of Medicine, 372(9), 793-795.

Additional References for Further Reading

- Harvard Medical School. (2023). Precision Medicine and Genetics in Healthcare.
- World Health Organization (WHO). (2022). Genomics and Health.
- National Institutes of Health (NIH). (2023). Genetic and Rare Diseases Information Center (GARD).